The Science
of
Ageing Backward

ReGeneration-X

Roderick Lane, Elizabeth Bright

Illustrations by Emalia Mattia

DEDICATION

Welcome to The Science of Ageing Backwards- ReGeneration-X.
This book is part of a series that deals with fundamental health issues
and aims to guide you through a eating pattern that sustains vitality
and health while reducing the need of 'age related medication'.

We walk in the footsteps of ancient mankind.

This book is dedicated to Generation-X and Generation-A those
first 200 individuals who walked out of the wilderness of Africa to
populate the rest of the world. The life style they followed, fasting
and feasting, ketogenic and paleolithic enabled the world as we know
it to be produced. While they were probably unaware of it, their life
style and dietary eating pattern produced in them a fundamental
health and vitality that is now lost in our society.

This book helps you reproduce the health that was enjoyed by
Generation-A. Walk alongside your ancestors and view the world
through the eyes of early man and explore your own new continent
of health.

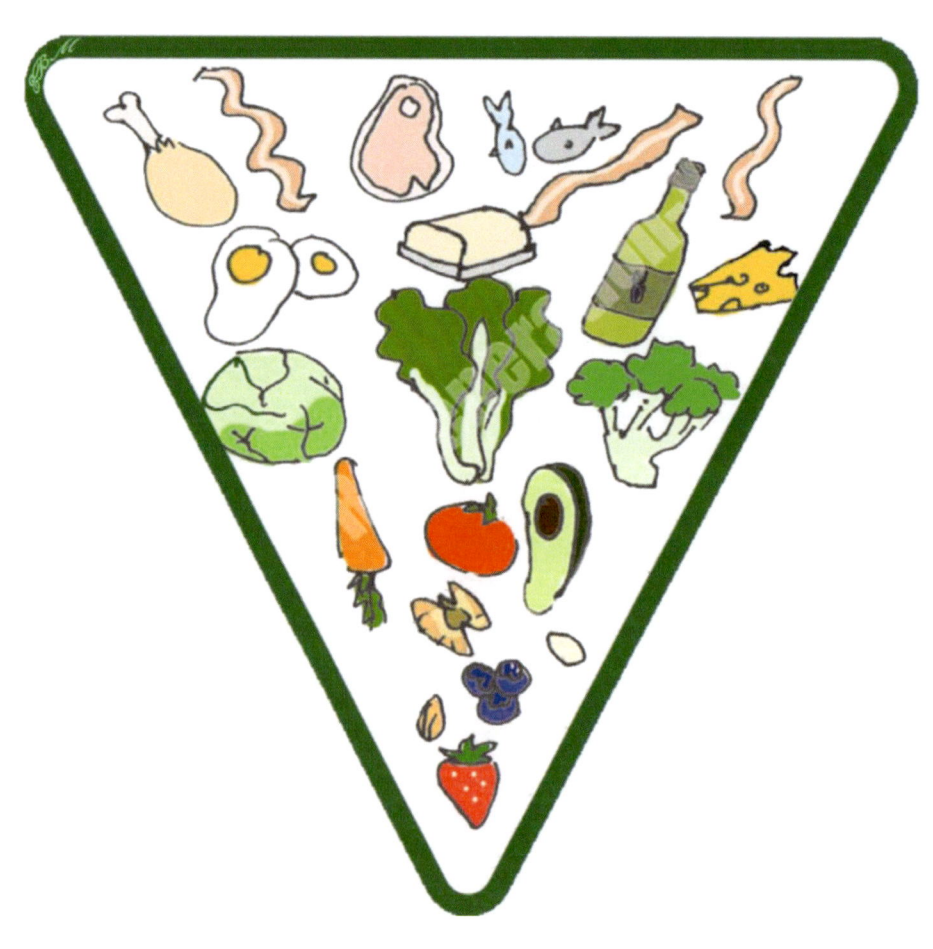

The ketogenic peoples

Let's take a short walk through the history of humanity, our dietary development, and the role of ketogenesis in humankind's survival and development.

There are no absolutes in mankind's dietary requirement. We have developed the unique ability to pretty much eat anything we come across and see. In reality we now eat far fewer foods than our predecessors. Our predecessors were adaptive beings. They developed stone tools and learned to hunt animals that were far more effective hunters and far more intimidating than we are.

It is often remarked that early man's life was 'short, nasty and brutal'. But was it? If life is so brutal you stay in the areas you know because food supply is predictable. You would not have time to explore. Neither would you have time to carve ornaments, make bead necklaces, perfect the art of tattooing, and paint beautiful murals on the inside walls of caves. Innovation would be a waste of hunting and gathering time. Conservatism is not a political statement when survival is the priority, it's the concept of 'do what you understand and works, or die'.

We know from studies conducted on rats and mice that underfed animals live longer, are more active, and suffer far less clinical disease than those fed the calorific 'norm'. Therefore the 'short' aspect of life is probably not true. Studies of societies that were still hunting and eating foods direct from their environment have shown that the average lifespan was similar to that which we have achieved in Europe today. Victorian man lived a shorter life than the American Indian. The native American existed on a lower starch-based calorific intake and was subject to seasonal low carbohydrate-based calorie fluctuations.

A study conducted in the 1970s in South Africa shows that even at times of catastrophic harvest failure, hunter-gatherer units were not impacted. During the 70s, for three years running, the agrarian peoples living in close proximity to the Bushmen of the Kalahari suffered catastrophic crop failure to the extent that the WHO declared an emergency and was supplying food aid. This failure did not affect the bushmen. The women were still gleaning foods, and found enough for three days' supply for every working day spent gathering. The male hunters changed techniques and practices to consume what was in abundance. One of the interesting observations from the bushmen point of view is that 'All game now concentrates on the water holes so hunting is now easier'.

This brings us to an interesting speculation: a species that thrives at the point of catastrophic failure will emerge as the dominant hunter and can continue expansion of its genetic stock. However, due to the increase of carbohydrates in the diet, i.e. refined flours and sugars, and the elimination of saturated fats for the last three decades, the descendants of the once-healthy hunter-gatherer species will suffer from the long list of degenerative "modern diseases" in spite of their resilient genetics.

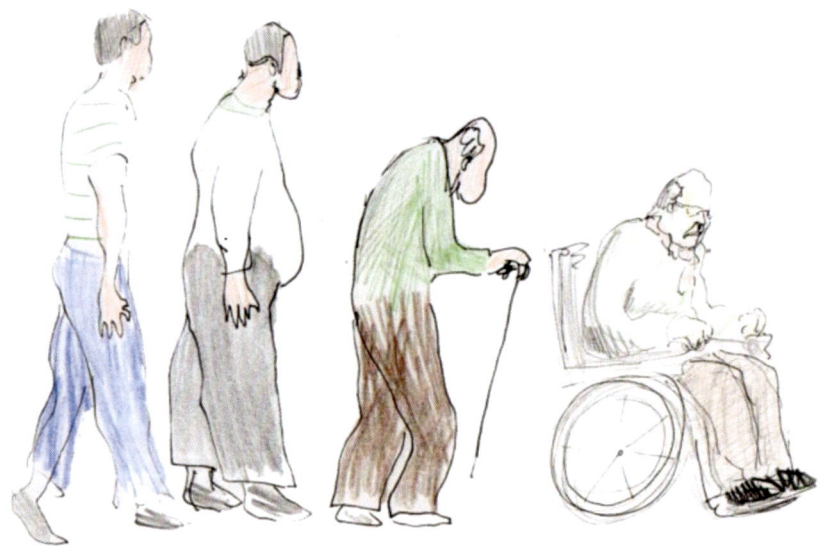

Don't degenerate, age backward - REGENERATE!

The low-starch diet changes and creates a healthy blood-lipid profile. HDL goes up, LDL goes down, and the LDL 'A' and 'B' ratio becomes predominantly 'A' fraction. 'A' fraction LDL is biochemically useful and does not cause arterial plaque. Most people, including many GP's, are unaware that there are two kinds of LDL — cholesterol 'A' (big and fluffy, easy to break down) and 'B' (small, dense and very nasty). 'B' fraction rises with the consumption of starches and sugars. Most importantly, the insulin levels would have been very stable on a low-starch diet, which would increase endurance, mental clarity, and give a general sense of well-being. Stable insulin implies no insulin resistance or increase of oxidative stress and cell death. I think a hunter-gatherer camp at the point of ketogenesis would have been a pretty jolly place to live. Imagine a place with little or no depression. If there were depressives, the depression was treated with rituals that would be life-affirming. In this place there was no clinical degenerative disease and people were capable of fending for themselves and contributing to their society well into their 90's. This created a social cohesion that had no concept of not-helping. A pretty easy life, in fact.

For mankind, with the advent of such things as the sling, bolas and atlatl (long-range spear-based weapon that can readily impart to a projectile speeds of over 150 km/h (93 mph), the nature of survival changed radically. With atlatls, mankind became the ultimate predator, and given that it was a device of skill rather than muscular force, it could be used by women and children with ease. A group of roving humans would be an incredibly formidable group. With the advent of this 'high- powered rifle' or a weapon of similar skill, such as the sling and bolas, mankind could rove. The ability to hunt from a distance increased safety and raised the amount of game that could be caught; it also made small migratory units possible and more viable; mankind no longer moved in herds but in packs. Consider it similar to going from the massed ranks of Napoleonic troops marching and migrating in thousands, down to small highly-efficient Special Forces units that are independent and can move quickly and efficiently. With the advent of things you can throw with force and with ease, the migratory pattern, the potential for survival and success goes off the scale.

So in essence we go from…

Yea, though I walk through the valley of the shadow of death, I will fear no evil: for thou art with me; thy rod and thy staff they comfort me.

To quote the biker badge we go to
Yea, though I walk through the valley of the shadow of death, I will fear no evil: for I am the meanest son of a bitch in the entire valley!

The hunter-gatherer lifestyle is a far more complex set of biochemical and physiological reactions than modern man has ever considered. It is primarily a low-glycemic, high-fat, moderate-protein lifestyle that is rich in densely packed nutrients taken from berries, herbs and fresh greens. The high-fat nutrients, which made up most of the calories in the hunter-gatherer diet, were packed with energy, double the energy coming from protein and carbohydrates. The moderate amount of protein was enough to rebuild and regenerate connective tissue, such as muscles and bones needed for running and hunting. There were no gyms taking the place of the hunting and gathering necessary for survival. With little or no glucose in their diet, they burnt all of it. Little energy was spent in enzymatically breaking down carbohydrates, thus saving the vital organs time and energy. No fat was stored, all systems ran smoothly. The hunter-gatherer suffered more from acute health problems, such as losing a leg to a tiger or bear, than the chronic diseases that are born of physiological systems out of balance. This lifestyle and pattern of eating would change from continent to continent depending on the availability and accessibility of starches, game and fish. In reality there would be a different form of hunter-gatherer diet for every continent and every particular area of human habitation.

The key factor all these early mankind diets share is fasting and feasting. At this point we must define the meaning of the word fast. Wikipedia defines fast as primarily an act of willing abstinence or reduction from certain or all food, drink, or both for a period of time. An absolute fast is normally defined as abstinence from all food and liquid for a defined period, usually a single day (24 hours), or several days. Other fasts may be only partially restrictive, limiting particular foods or substances. The fast may also be intermittent in nature.

A true fast in Western medical terms is one where only water is consumed. A fast is not a mono diet, when one is only living on fruit juice (which is very high in sugars), brown beans, or grapes. A true fast for 24 hours pushes an individual into ketogenesis, that is, the burning of stored body fat to produce ketones. Ketones are a naturally occurring energy source. At this point I must emphasize that ketone production is natural; most people awake in the morning with an elevated ketone level because they have not eaten all night, hence the name for breakfast. A controlled elevated ketone level must not be confused with Ketoacidosis, which is a clinical side effect of poor blood sugar management often found in diabetics.

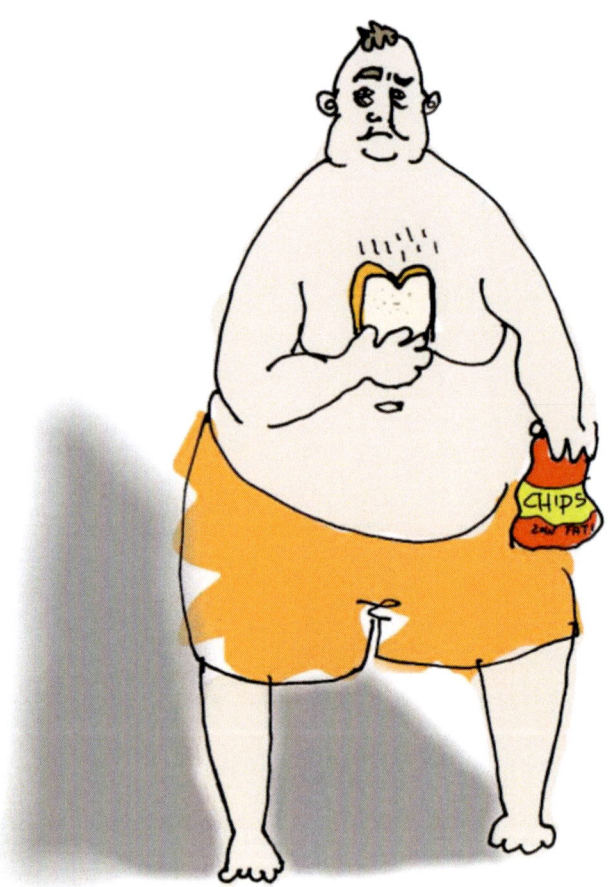

The food we eat

It may come as no surprise to many people that the very nature of the food we eat these days has fundamentally changed. If you take something as commonplace as the humble banana and look at the wild variety, you will see an amazing difference. The wild variety is small, very stringy, full of seeds, and would take you about an hour to chew through. The modern domesticated banana — I use the term modern loosely - is a starch and sugar-rich food which has about 30 times more carbohydrates than its primitive ancestor. Hunter-gatherer man did eat bananas, but the banana of that era contained more fiber and seeds than an entire can of modern laxatives!

Genetic manipulation has been going on since man began to plant and farm crops. Our farmer ancestors were able to coax natural variants they found in plants to produce a higher starch content. But this was a natural form of genetic manipulation, relying upon the plant's natural survival technique. Man learned to nurture natural evolutionary changes, such as in South America, where the Inca grew both white and green cotton, having found green cotton — a natural mutation — in the fields. Man's ability to nurture nature is different from synthetic genetic manipulation.

The food we ate

Persistence hunting is a technique in which hunters use a combination of running, walking, and tracking to pursue prey to the point of exhaustion. While humans can sweat to reduce body heat, their quadrupedal prey would need to slow from a gallop in order to pant. In his many lectures and writings, Sir Laurens Jan van der Post describes this process of hunting, having witnessed it first hand. Today, persistence hunting is very rare and seen only in a few groups such as Kalahari bushmen and the Tarahumara or Raramuri people of Northern Mexico. The technique requires endurance running – running long distances for extended periods of time - and among primates, endurance running is only seen in humans. Persistence hunting is thought to have been one of the earliest forms of human hunting, having evolved 2 million years ago. The Lykov family of six are known for spending 42 years in complete isolation from human society in an otherwise uninhabited upland of the Abakan Range, in the Tashtypsky District of Khakassia (southern Siberia). It is believed that they reverted to persistence hunting in their isolation to gather food.

The key: Persistence and endurance
While man, with the advent of his new super weapons, was a formidable hunter, the basic form of hunting was persistence hunting. This means jogging along after an animal until that animal actually gives up due to exhaustion. Man and horses are the only two animals that actively sweat, man's sweating ability being greater than that of a horse. This ability enables us to cool ourselves when we are moving rapidly as compared to the animals that we have traditionally hunted, which have to stop and pant to cool down. So our ability to run long distances, or at least to maintain a moderate pace for long distances, enables us to catch game. If you're running after an animal like an antelope, you don't carry a rucksack containing everything from the kitchen sink to a new pair of shoes. If you're lucky you carry some water, because thirst will be your primary concern.

When you are persistence hunting there is no guarantee that you will actually catch your prey instantly; you may have to jog/run up to 25 miles before the animal in question gives up. Even then there is a chance that another predator might actually catch the animal, or that the prey will hide successfully in the undergrowth, and you have spent the entire day running after lunch which has successfully evaded you. Here we begin to see the value and the necessity of man's ability to go into ketosis; if you have not caught dinner you will be hungry, yet your body will still need nutrition and energy for the hunt for the next day. The obvious and economical physiological thing to do is to burn any of the body fat that you are carrying, and to use this body fat to feed cellular energy by the most direct method. Fats in the bloodstream (ketones) only need three enzymes in the human cell to produce energy. Sugars need 23 enzymes. In ketosis, the body is operating on a very direct and simple energy mechanism, but that's not where it ends.

Ketone energy is a very specific energy source for the human metabolism. Interestingly, it does not support nor feed aberrant tissue. That is, it is not a primary energy source or support for cancer. Cancer prefers sugar as its primary fuel. This leads to a very interesting observation — that early man whilst hunting continually slipped in and out of ketosis and this process would have had the effect of killing small clusters of cancerous cells, or at least denying them energy to thrive and replicate. It is also known that a ketogenic diet, if sustained, will strip arteries of cholesterol and arterial plaque, normalize blood cholesterol levels, and during the process of ketosis, reduce the need for insulin. Ketogenic diets in the past and at present have been used very successfully for controlling type II diabetes and also in some cases for correcting the onset of type I diabetes (Cantin Diet). Possibly the first recorded incident in modern times is the Banting diet (1797-1878) which was formulated by Dr. William Harvey.

Dr. Harvey had recently returned from a symposium in Paris where he had heard Dr. Claude Bernard, a renowned physiologist, talk of a new theory about the part played by the liver in the disease of diabetes. Bernard believed that the liver, in addition to secreting bile, also secreted a sugar-like substance that it made from elements of the blood passing through it. This started Harvey's thinking about the roles of the various food elements in diabetes and he began a major course of research into the question of how fats, sugars and starches affect the body. Harvey's advice to Banting was to give up bread, butter, milk, sugar, beer and potatoes. These, he told Banting, contained starch and saccharine matter tending to create fat and were to be avoided completely. The word 'saccharine' meant sugar.

And as they say, the rest is history. The Banting process has fallen in and out of favor and has been marketed under several different names since the 1800s. We are now at a point where medical science is actually looking at the value of ketosis and ketones with a purely scientific eye rather than an eye that has been corrupted by misinformation and poor science. All the past and future variants of the Banting diet have had one thing in common: ketosis.

Calories in, calories out, old science. Fat in, fat out, with modern proven clinical testing.

The key to health is to re-engage with the fundamental lost 'cellular muscle' ketosis. This alternative, naturally occurring, and available energy supply enables insulin function, adrenal function, and allows much of the endocrine system to relax and regenerate. In essence ketosis, if it is used routinely, is a method by which the body can rest its own internal mechanisms while maintaining health, energy and energetic function.

Ketosis, the simple biochemical tool that enabled early man to survive and to thrive.

Ketosis, the simple biochemical tool that enabled man to run and hunt.

Ketosis, the simple biochemical state that reduced inflammation and refused to feed cancer.

Ketosis, the lost cellular muscle of endurance and energy.

Before we get into the dos and don'ts of following a ketogenic diet, it's very important that you establish what it is you wish to achieve. The concept of 'I just want to lose weight' is not enough.

The action of ReGeneration-X is to turn back the clock and get you to a point in your personal history and memory that you remember as being full of health and vitality. In turning back the clock you should have certain goals and aims. Below is a basic checklist of some of the things you can ask yourself.

Do you want to..?
lose weight
change body shape
normalize cholesterol
increase lung volume
be happier
control moods
normalize blood sugar levels
fit into wedding suit/dress or fit into that dress/pair of jeans you saved from your thinner days
be able to walk up staircase
run a marathon
climb a mountain
ride a bicycle
dance the tango

walk the coastal path

And then there are unwanted results of inappropriate eating and diet..

Do you..?
1. get routinely angry when you are hungry?
2. have brain fog?
3. go more than three hours without craving coffee or eating?
4. have enough energy to last you through the day?
5. wake up in the middle of the night hungry?
6. get headaches during the day?
7. feel as if you need to go to sleep during the afternoon?
8. feel so exhausted after exercising that you suffer acute nausea?
9. exercise without eating?
10. need to immediately have something sweet like an energy drink after you exercise?

As you can see when you begin to work on your list, the benefit of the ketogenic diet begins to expand across your entire life. Many of the things you may have considered inevitable, or were told were usual 'given your age', are in fact not. The concept of 'given your age' is an entirely spurious one. We all know and have met people who are doing fantastically well for reasons of their own. Neither is good fundamental health financially related. The wealthy end up in wheelchairs just as do the poor. Your health is often down to your own dietary choices and this fundamental choice has nothing to do with social strata but it has an awful lot to do with desire and common sense. The answer to the old phrase which asks 'if this is common sense, why isn't everyone else doing it?'

You are! The fact that you are reading this proves that you have uncommon good sense! You are part of a unique group in our society who have decided not to live on medication or just suffer from it because it happens 'given your age'. Rather you have voted with your feet, or in this case your stomach, and decided to do something about your life and kick down the hospital doors.

I'm going to run a few concepts by you which, when you think about them, actually are uncommon common sense. Lots of people assume that they are not eating sugars, but they are eating complex carbohydrates. What they are not familiar with is that complex carbohydrates contained in root vegetables, whole grains, and general health foods are in fact long chains of glucose molecules. The digestion does what it always does with long chains of glucose molecules. It breaks them down into smaller chains i.e. sugars which then impact on the bloodstream and the body as though you were consuming refined sugar. So remember the next time you pick up that whole-earth, full-grain, organic, biodynamic guaranteed dried fruit natural nutrition bar — all you are doing is eating a rather big block of very expensive sugar! And here's another caution — just because something is vegetarian, organic or planet-friendly, does not make it sugar-free. Often the low-fat bars have the highest obvious and hidden sugar content around.

If you're a pet owner you will be familiar with this question. When you take your animal in for an examination by the veterinary surgeon, the first question the veterinarian will ask is 'what foods are you feeding your pet'? Veterinary surgeons are taught, and have long since worked out, that what you feed a domestic animal greatly affects its health. If your vet is not hooked into some trading mechanism associated with an incredibly expensive dried animal food, they inevitably say 'well, try feeding this animal a little raw meat (not advised for goldfish) as its digestive tract is actually designed for non-cooked foods'. In truth you are what you eat, digest, process, utilize and excrete.

The science and knowledge of fat building and fat burning has changed radically since the 1970's. Our understanding is now closer to that of physicians from 150 years ago.

Here is an even more bizarre fact. In 1979 a horse called No Bombs won a race at Royal Ascot Race Course, but was disqualified when traces of stimulant showed up in a post-race test. The horse's owners, managers and trainers were mystified - until it emerged that No Bombs had stolen and eaten a stable-lad's Mars bar (chocolate toffee bar) shortly before the race. The chocolate contained caffeine and theobromine, two mild stimulants which are banned in horse racing, and the disqualification stood. Still think food does not affect your biochemistry?

Put another way, if you owned an aircraft and an engineer asked if you are maintaining it properly, and your answer was "yes, I do the normal things that are recommended." Do you think an engineer would accept that? You are infinitely more sophisticated than a 747 jet, yet the engineer who is supposed to look after you never asks you what your actual maintenance schedule is, i.e. what are you eating, when are you eating it, and what are you putting into what you are eating. If you think of yourself as an aircraft and then consider the lack of supervision that you have been subject to, I'm pretty sure you'd never climb on board and try and reach for the sky. Remember the junk food, sugars and hidden sugars you put in your body are inevitably not utilized. They just go into fat storage and gather metabolic dust. When you are in permanent fat storage you actually have to carry them around, and that's mentally, emotionally, physically and psychologically exhausting.

Some of the benefits you gain from this dietary system will not be instantly obvious when you consider the amount of years that we have all been consuming, often in good faith, foods packed with pesticides, monosodium glutamate, fructose and food dyes. We can remember when such things as DDT were sprayed in houses, although now it is known to have been one of the most polluting and poisonous substances on the planet. For a lifetime we have been consuming and been subjected to foods that are in fact endocrine disruptors, that is, they mimic hormones and also play havoc with what hormones are supposed to do naturally. Man is an adaptive animal and we adapt to how we are eating, but that adaption comes at a cost. High sugar/carbohydrate diets, which have been literally forced down our throats for the last 60 years, are taking us down a path where we are all becoming predisposed to clinical obesity, clogged arteries and diabetes.

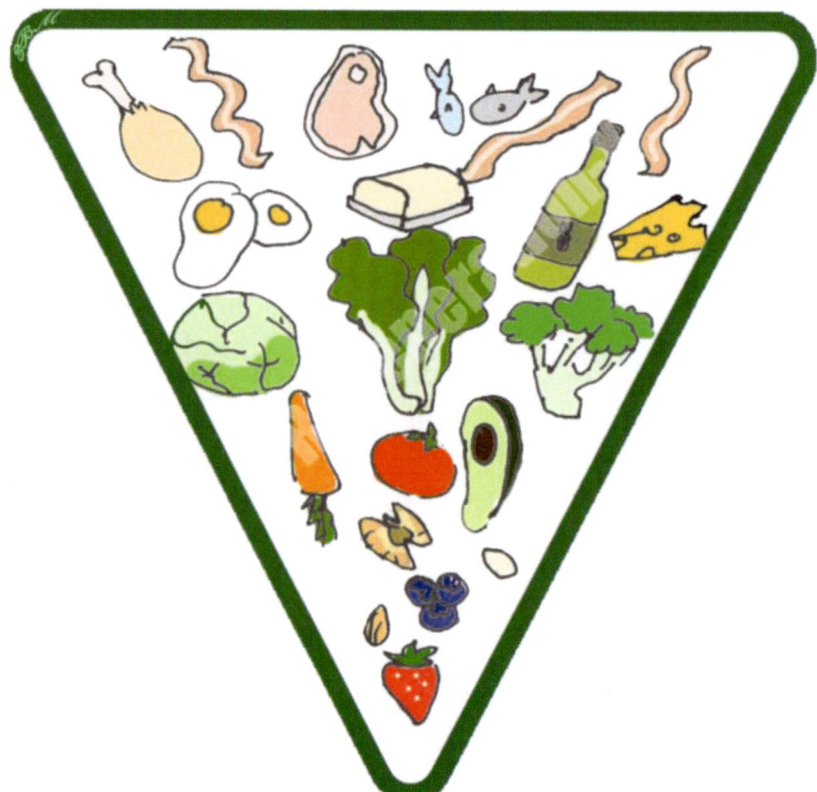

The ReGeneration-X food Triangle

This, within a modern context, is the manner in which our ancestors formerly ate. We say the modern context because in our society foods, like people, have emigrated; maize is now in Europe and cows are now in the Americas. Many of the advocates of 'paleo diets' and vegetarian diets forget that they are using a very broad spectrum of foods that 500 years ago would not have been found together or associated. In truth the paleo choices from country to country would have been far more limited.

Drugs and pharmaceuticals

Do you go to the pharmacy with a pile of prescriptions for medications which you know may possibly hurt you in the long run? The ketogenic diet has the potential to replace those drugs by improving the conditions for which many pharmaceuticals are prescribed, from diabetes to hypertension, without the scary side-effects.

We have taken this information from the UK National Health Service as it is a centralized system and all medications in the UK are dispensed as part of the NHS. The UK system is government-organized and not based on private subscriptions or insurance; the figures it provides are therefore fairly accurate. The UK prescribes at a fairly conservative rate compared to the USA; these numbers are based on a population of 65 million. This implies that over half the population are on cholesterol-lowering drugs now known to be less than perfect and having critical side-effects for many. 1

Cardiovascular therapies dominate generic-prescribing in England, figures from the NHS Information Centre show. Drugs for cardiovascular disease (CVD) take four of the five highest places among the top 10 most prescribed generic drugs. The thyroid treatment (levothyroxine sodium) is the only non-CVD treatment among the top five places. Numbers of prescriptions for two proton-pump inhibitors (lansoprazole and omeprazole) are almost equal and scrape into the tail-end of the top 10, though if combined these two would be among the top three most prescribed generic drugs.

Let's start with the cholesterol-lowering drugs, the statins.

1. Simvastatin, 37.3 million prescribed.
Simvastatin is used along with a proper diet to help lower cholesterol and fats (such as LDL, triglycerides) and raise "good" cholesterol (HDL) in the blood. It belongs to a group of drugs known as "statins." It works by reducing the amount of cholesterol made by the liver. Since this statement entered the public domain it has now been demonstrated that they are very inefficient, almost bordering on useless, yet poor ratios of LDL A and B cholesterols still remain an issue.

2. Aspirin, 33.9 million prescribed
Aspirin "thins" the blood and helps prevent blood clots from forming, hence it helps prevent heart attack and stroke. There is a risk of stomach problems, including stomach bleeding, for people

who take aspirin regularly.

3. Levothyroxine sodium, 21.9 million

Levothyroxine is used to treat an underactive thyroid (hypothyroidism). It replaces or provides more thyroid hormone, which is normally produced by the thyroid gland. Low thyroid-hormone levels can occur naturally or when the thyroid gland is injured by radiation/medications or removed by surgery.

4. Ramipril 19.3 million

Ramipril (Altace) is an ACE inhibitor. ACE stands for angiotension converting enzyme. Ramipril is used to treat high blood pressure (hypertension) or congestive heart failure, and to improve survival after a heart attack.

5. Bendroflumethiazide 18.8 million

Bendroflumethiazide tablets belong to a group of medicines called thiazide diuretics (water tablets). They may be used to reduce fluid retention (edema) particularly in the heart, kidneys, liver or that caused by medication, by increasing the flow of urine and reduce high blood pressure alone or with other medication.

6. Paracetamol 18.8 million

Paracetamol (acetaminophen) is a pain reliever and a fever reducer. The exact mechanism of action is not known. Paracetamol is used to treat many conditions such as headache, muscle aches, arthritis, backache, toothaches, colds, and fevers.

7. Salbutamol 18.7 million

Salbutamol (Albuterol) is used to treat or prevent bronchospasm in patients with asthma, bronchitis, emphysema, and other lung diseases. This medicine is also used to prevent wheezing caused by exercise (exercise-induced bronchospasm).

8. Omeprazole 18.3 million

Omeprazole (Prilosec, Zegerid) belongs to a group of drugs called proton pump inhibitors. It decreases the amount of acid produced in the stomach. Omeprazole is used to treat symptoms of gastroesophageal reflux disease (GERD) and other conditions caused by excess stomach acid.

9. Lansoprazole 14.9 million
Lansoprazole is used to treat and prevent stomach and intestinal ulcers, erosive esophagitis (damage to the esophagus from stomach acid), and other conditions involving excessive stomach acid such as Zollinger-Ellison syndrome (a condition in which a gastrin-secreting tumor or hyperplasia of the islet cells in the pancreas cause overproduction of gastric acid, resulting in recurrent peptic ulcers).

10. Co-codamol 14.6 million
It consists of a mixture of paracetamol plus codeine phosphate (a member of the class of drugs called opioid analgesics). In general, co-codamol is used as required to relieve mild-to-moderate pain and to reduce fever, and so is used for the relief of headaches, migraine, toothache, back pain and period pains.

Cholesterol-lowering drugs or the alternative

Below is one of the many studies that support the use of a ketogenic diet. It was not done by us and does not reflect our bias or enthusiasm for the subject. You will note that it mentions good reactions and positive changes for all of the conditions associated with the drugs listed above.

The present study shows the beneficial effects of a long-term ketogenic diet. It significantly reduced the body weight and body mass index of the patients. Furthermore, it decreased the level of triglycerides, LDL cholesterol and blood glucose, and increased the level of HDL cholesterol. Administering a ketogenic diet for a relatively longer period of time did not produce any significant side effects in the patients. Therefore, the present study confirms that it is safe to use a ketogenic diet for a longer period of time than previously demonstrated. You will find a link to the full study in our notes section.2

Long-term effects of a ketogenic diet in obese patients.
Dashti HM, Mathew TC, Hussein T, Asfar SK, Behbahani A, Khourseed MA, Al-Sayer HM, Bo-Abbas YY, Al-Zaid NS.
KEYWORDS: Diet; Ketosis; Obesity
SOURCE: PubMed

OBJECTIVE:
To determine the effects of a 24-week ketogenic diet (consisting of 30 g carbohydrate, 1 g/kg body weight protein, 20% saturated fat, and 80% polyunsaturated and monounsaturated fat) in obese patients.

PATIENTS AND METHODS:
In the present study, 83 obese patients (39 men and 44 women) with a body mass index greater than 35 kg/m(2), and high glucose and cholesterol levels were selected. The body weight, body mass index, total cholesterol, low density lipoprotein (LDL) cholesterol, high density lipoprotein (HDL) cholesterol, triglycerides, fasting blood sugar, urea and creatinine levels were determined before and after the administration of the ketogenic diet. Changes in these parameters were monitored after eight, 16 and 24 weeks of treatment.

RESULTS:
The weight and body mass index of the patients decreased significantly (P<0.0001). The level of total cholesterol decreased from week 1 to week 24. HDL cholesterol levels significantly increased, whereas LDL cholesterol levels significantly decreased after treatment. The level of triglycerides decreased significantly following 24 weeks of treatment. The level of blood glucose significantly decreased. The changes in the level of urea and creatinine were not statistically significant.

CONCLUSIONS:
The present study shows the beneficial effects of a long-term ketogenic diet. It significantly reduced the body weight and body mass index of the patients. Furthermore, it decreased the level of triglycerides, LDL cholesterol and blood glucose, and increased the level of HDL cholesterol. Administering a ketogenic diet for a relatively longer period of time did not produce any significant side effects in the patients. Therefore, the present study confirms that it is safe to use a ketogenic diet for a longer period of time than previously demonstrated.

Commentary
This is one of the many clinical studies found on the internet conducted by recognized medical researchers. The total blood lipid profile fell and the good cholesterol ration increased while the bad cholesterol decreased. In addition, they all lost weight and blood

glucose levels stabilized. For an individual who is a type 2 diabetic, obese and on cholesterol medication this 24-week diet, supported by orthodox medical evidence, makes common sense.

Consider this, possibly 30 million of those prescriptions are not needed or even necessary. The savings to the NHS or an individual's pocket could be immense.

Adapting to the diet

One of the first acts of many people is to take a proposed new diet and wave it under the nose of your doctor and demand 'what do you think?' Many doctors are aware of ketogenics and use it for their own health and vitality, but they are often very reluctant to prescribe it for a client. Why?

Doctors are in a peculiar position where if they do not tell you to take statins or do a low fat diet they are not following the 'advice' of their peer group. In spite of the fact that they know statins are useless and that also low fat diets don't work (if they did you would be a lean, mean fighting machine already) and that there is pure scientific evidence and fact going back to the 1800's demonstrating that ketogenics do work as a life style. The doctor's greatest fear is that while you are standing in line a meteor falls from the sky and knocks you off your feet, some enterprising lawyer will then sue him for having placed you on a 'non approved medical diet'. If you were not on that diet and still walking with a stick you would not have made it to the line, so it's the doctor's fault that you were hit by the meteor. Joking aside this is pretty much the case, people tend to blame others for their own mistakes and negligence.

The Adaptation Phase

Moving into ketogenesis (fat burning) from glucogenesis (sugar burning), or swapping the fuel sources around, will take a toll on some. Many have become so glucose-dependent that they go through withdrawal symptoms as the biochemistry adapts.

Contrary to the popular belief, the process of a ketogenic diet is not all holistic medicine, organic, pure and life-affirming. The ketogenic diet is actually a clinical tool just like a spanner, a pair of scissors or spellcheck when used when writing a document on a computer. The ketogenic diet is not perfect (nor is any specific diet), but it is generally easy to do and very well-tolerated by most adults and adolescents. There are reported side-effects from people who have been on extreme ketogenic diets of slightly elevated cholesterol, but this is not something to worry about as it is in fact the good cholesterol level which rises and the bad cholesterol level which falls. Constipation is reported, but this is usually only reported in those who are not drinking enough water, or whose intestines are adjusting to the changes in their intestinal flora. Without carbohydrates, some bacteria and fungi that colonized the intestine to digest and feed off carbohydrates, such as candida, will die, and this is a good thing. The same can be said for the reports of kidney stones. It has been observed by natural practitioners for many generations that those who do not drink adequate water tend to develop kidney stones. Reports of constipation may also be due to the cultural avoidance of fats. Fats, such as coconut oil and lard, which are increased on the ketogenic diet, have a laxative effect.

The withdrawal symptoms, which in my experience are proportional to how long you have been overweight and how long you have been starch-dependent, happen to about 10% of people. In essence, your withdrawal state indicates how badly maladapted your biochemistry has become.

The 10% may suffer from the following:
Weakness
Fatigue
Nausea
Dehydration and increased urination
Diarrhea
Constipation
Dizziness and or Orthostatic hypotension (if you stand up quickly your blood pressure drops)
Gout symptoms if you already have the problem.

Don't Panic!

These effects are all known to be short-term and you are in this for the long-term (outlive your doctor and bank manager etc.). These are symptoms of carbohydrate withdrawal, some people panic and start back on the carbohydrates, but this is the equivalent of telling a drug addict that to stop the pains, 'hit the drugs man, they will make you feel better!' This of course is a ridiculous statement to make, but it illustrates the point: all the scientific evidence, experience and articles lead us to understand that the long-term benefits outweigh the short term downsides. If you want a lean body, clear mind, clean arteries, a drug-free existence and the ability to run when others hobble: keto adapt.

'Carb withdrawal' symptoms have very little to do with the high-fat content of the diet, they are mainly due to poor management and old dietary habits creeping in, i.e. 'I will do high-protein but cut down on the fats — fats are nasty everyone knows that.'

One of the things we have mentioned before is the ability of a ketogenic diet to stabilize endocrine-system fluctuations. The main culprit involved in these fluctuations is insulin. In response to carbohydrate-forced insulin surges we can develop all manner of conditions, including diabetes, insulin resistance, hypothyroidism, high blood pressure, cortisol resistance etc, etc. Insulin is the hidden trigger.

<u>Insulin can push starches and sugars into the fat cells, as the more insulin you promote the more you feed your fat cells.</u>

Anyone who's ever tried a lifestyle-change will have come to the conclusion that fat cells pretty much have a mind of their own. It seems not to matter what we do because the fat cell always wins. Inevitably it wins because it is an intimate part of our natural energy and survival strategy. It's just that the fat cell is being triggered continually in the wrong manner by insulin surges. Insulin is necessary for our survival but probably in far less concentration than we are normally subjected to in this current environment of high refined-carbohydrate diets.

Insulin does the following things:

1. In the fat cell it turns on the lipoprotein lipase enzyme. The LPL is essentially a little hook that sits on the outside of your fat cells; when stimulated by insulin it catches fat and pushes fat into storage in the fat cells.
2. Inside the fat cell, insulin turns off hormone-sensitive lipase. HSL is responsible for liberating stored fat from the fat cell. It's involved in the biochemical process of breaking down the stored fat into its component fatty-acid parts and releasing them into the bloodstream to be used as cellular fuel.
3. Insulin is incredibly sensitive to any shift in blood sugar. Even a small amount of carbohydrate or sugar release will stimulate insulin's role as a hormonal modulator. Anything that increases insulin levels increases the amount of fat storage.

To put this simply, the events that lead to the increased storage of body fat, and more importantly to stop the body fat from being released for essential energy, are as follows:

1. You eat something containing carbohydrate. This applies to whatever carbohydrate base you eat whether it be refined carbohydrate or complex carbohydrate; in essence, any form of sugar.
2. The consequence of eating is that you begin to secrete insulin.
3. The release of insulin into your bloodstream increases uptake of stored fat and shuts down the release of fats for energy.
4. As the meal is digested and more carbohydrates enter into your bloodstream, your blood sugar levels elevate.
5. In response to this further increase of circulating carbohydrates, you secrete more insulin.
6. The increase of insulin shuts down the HSL, further preventing any release of fats for energy consumption.
7. This cycle continues until there are no more carbohydrates in the bloodstream and the insulin level drops.

This happens not only when you consume carbohydrate-based foods; it also happens when you consume protein. The body metabolizes what it needs from the amino acids in protein for connective tissue. Any excess is metabolized as a glucose. That is why when you consume a high-fat, moderate-protein meal there is no secondary insulin response as very little sugar/carbohydrates circulate in your bloodstream. So the action of insulin becomes very mild compared to the massive insulin rush which many people with low blood sugar (hypoglycemia) will have experienced when insulin kicks in and drops their blood sugar level radically.

Some protein foods are insulinogenic, such as nuts and dairy, and may provoke a higher insulin reaction, so it is best to avoid these at the beginning of the diet. In these days of drinks-beverages, snacks and 'naughty but nice' cakes and cookies it is quite easy to see why it is virtually impossible for many to lose weight. Add to this that a lifetime exposure to these fast-acting sugars can create a process of insulin resistance (the body becomes less responsive to insulin) and we have a recipe for disaster. In insulin resistance the reaction of the human body is to pump out even more insulin, and this greater flood of insulin produces even more fat storage.

The rather peculiar thing about this is that our biochemistry eventually becomes adapted to feeding the fat cells but not providing you with fundamental energy. One of the great things about ketogenics is that by going into ketosis we shut down to a greater extent the insulin mechanism, and give all of our biochemistry a chance to basically reset, rest, and reboot. This fundamental alternative-energy mechanism is a useful tool that allows our biochemistry to mend itself at the most fundamental level.

The bottom line is, the more we stimulate insulin production via junk food, sodas, fruit juices, pastries, cookies, french fries and pizza, the less we enable our body to utilize stored fats for energy. The good news is that on ketogenics you don't feel hungry because you're feeding the cells, not the fat-storage mechanism.

Things to do

Dehydration and urination: Ensure you have an adequate salt intake, sodium enables you to retain potassium. Do not follow a low-salt diet on ketogenics. This will help mass urination problems. Use sea salt, celtic salt and bone broth.

Constipation: Drink water, not tea, coffee, herb tea etc. Are you eating too much protein in relation to fat?

Weakness and fatigue: Don't exercise. Adapt to the diet first before you fall into the exercise trap. Check your salt intake.

Nausea and Dizziness: Check salt and protein to fat ratio.
Gout: Hydration

Diarrhea: Excess protein, also can be a sign that your body is shedding residual drugs.

But my cholesterol went up!

Don't panic, your blood stream transports fats from storage to cells for energy to be converted and burned. Elevated blood fats is an initial ketogenic indicator of increased transport and burning. Eventually the levels drop. After all, if you wanted to dispose of 20kg of garbage from storage, you would put it in a sack and move it through the corridors and out of the house. At the point of moving, your 'house garbage level' would have risen, just like your cholesterol. After you have gotten rid of it all, your total level would drop.

Like any diet, the ketogenic diet requires work and commitment. One of the best things to do is to actually get yourself a 'diet buddy.' Weight Watchers was formed by a group of ladies sitting round a table giving each other mutual support while they were on their specific diets. Having a friend to gripe to and also support you makes the difference. Give yourself a 12-week commitment to the diet; you will find that after 12 weeks you have established a working habit. 12 weeks for anything is a very reasonable goal.

The 12 weeks allows you to fine-tune it and adapt it to your particular needs and lifestyle. Fine-tuning may require tinkering with the ratio of fat to protein, for the reasons mentioned above, due to insulin resistance or carbohydrate sensitivity. But benefits will be huge in a 12-week period.

In some cases with specific metabolic inhibitions or higher degree of toxicity, this might take longer. Those who have developed a high degree of insulin-resistance due to diet, age, stress or familial history of diabetes may require a longer period of adaptation. The same can apply to those with cortisol resistance which often go hand in hand with insulin resistance.

<u>The secret to adapting the diet to you: start with more fat, NOT less!</u>

One of the great things about having a diet buddy is that you can actually rant at each other and let off steam and they will know exactly why you are doing it. It's amazing how unsupportive partners and family can be when they don't understand what you're trying to achieve. A diet buddy is a great person to have on your side. Your family and friends are also caught in the 'oh you should expect that at your age' and the other famous comment of 'you should just eat less and exercise more!' Everyone has tried that and surprise, surprise, it does not work for 90% of humanity. For those for whom coping with the hunger pangs is a brutal exercise.

There will be some people who will be very doubtful and the word ketogenic will immediately ring little alarm bells in their heads because the ketogenic diet is often associated with the word ketoacidosis. Ketogenic is not, I repeat, not ketoacidosis.

Ketoacidosis primarily occurs in diabetics, as it is the inability to process and utilize glucose, which leads to inordinately high glucose levels accompanied by clinical dehydration. This in turn produces chemical imbalance and ketoacidosis.

Left untreated in a diabetic, this clinical case can lead to coma and sometimes even to death. This state of high glucose cannot occur in ketosis, the state you are in when you have adapted to the ketogenic diet, because on the ketogenic diet you are lowering your glucose level; hence, effects do not occur when someone is on the ketogenic diet. The ketogenic diet is a state of starvation, or glucose-restricted. However, ketoacidosis is an incredibly simple thing to treat in the non-diabetic, healthy individual with a glass of fresh orange juice. Ketoacidosis will go away in a healthy individual.

<u>Ketosis is NOT the same as ketoacidosis, a burning match is not a house fire.</u>

The ketogenic diet is a very old medical tool. It was used during the 20s and 30s in hospitals to help control, and in many cases, eliminate seizures and epilepsy. This diet has had a resurgence and is now used to treat childhood epilepsy for those who do not respond to the anti-convulsive drugs. I would caution you that this book is not a book for epileptics to control petit mal or grand mal seizure. The dietary process for the nutritional treatment of
these two problems, while similar to this, needs qualified medical intervention and observation.

Dr. Eric H. Kossoff, in his groundbreaking book Ketogenic Diets, mentions a case of a young man who had up to 70 epileptic seizures a day. After adopting a ketogenic diet the seizures went down to 5 a day within 24 hours, and after seven days the seizures stopped altogether. The power of ketones in many clinical conditions is often dramatic, made even more so by the fact that it's such a simple dietary change.

Measuring your ketones

Measuring your ketones is really quite simple. Once you have adopted the ketogenic diet, the ketones will be circulating freely in your bloodstream. Many of these ketones will be used for energy, but the excess will find their way into your urine; this excess can be measured with urinary dipsticks called ketostixs. You have to remember that ketones are essentially energy. If you have been running or working hard you may have burnt all available free ketones. During the night the liver works hard to produce glucose, gluconeogenesis, to make sure you have energy while you sleep, so if you test your urine in the morning you may actually be ketone-excess free. At this point don't be alarmed! This is just proof-positive that you are actually burning the ketones.

Eat a good high-fat, moderate-protein breakfast, and you will see that ketostix turn pink or purple. However, if you are getting decent ketone measurements on your ketostixs, these minor fluctuations in readings should not worry you. Just remember that what you find in your urine will not always correspond with what is going on in your bloodstream.

Consistent consumption of fat is the way to ensure ketosis. After 12 weeks you are keto-adapted. You may not need to measure your ketones, as the ketostix are only sensitive to acetoacetate, one of three ketones bodies. Ketostix are a cheap and easy way to confirm ketosis. After you are keto-adapted, you may only want to test your urine when and if you eat carbohydrates, and want to measure when you are again in ketosis.
When you are keto-adapted you convert more efficiently.

If you have food allergies and you find that a particular food is recommended in one of the recipes in this book, do the obvious thing and don't eat it! Unfortunately we cannot be there to watch over you and advise you, so using your not-so-common sense and your life experience is vital when undergoing a ketogenic diet. What we can say is that there are so many food options and things you can swap available on the market these days that food allergies should not be a problem with this diet.

Keep a food diary
"I do whatever it takes to get back my vitality and energy. The changes that I have committed to are worthwhile to have a wonderful life that is my right!'

Start off with this statement at the top of your food diary. If you start this process of regeneration with a positive attitude you will find it's very easy to do. Keeping a food diary may seem obvious, but it is crucial to know what you are eating, when you are eating it, and why you're eating it. Be honest in your food diary. From my own experience, until I kept a food diary, I always wondered why my ketone level dropped about lunchtime, then I realized that during my normal coffee break I usually ate a piece of fruit. I had never linked this with being a high-sugar consumption item, but it was. When I stopped eating the fruit my ketone levels went up and my body fat went down more quickly.

Foods

Double cream! One of the surprising things about the ketogenic diet is that you can actually have double cream! This is probably the most banned substance on all other diets known to man. Most double creams have between a 40% to 30% fat content; this content will vary from manufacturer to manufacturer and also may vary seasonally. Some pre-manufactured creams have added sugar. Even a single gram of additional sugar that sneaks into your diet from an unreliable source can take you out of ketosis. So watch the sugar count!

Food labeling

If you're using any form of pre-manufactured or processed food, read the label! Food manufacturers often change the protein, fat and sugar content of their products without any notice. The first thing you experience when coming out of ketosis is feeling sluggish again. Check online for particular foods that you eat, as many foods have very low levels of sugar which are not declared on the label. Checking online will enable you to calculate your sugar-loading correctly. There are also smartphone apps which allow you to scan bar codes for prepared foods. Remember it is always better, and you will see it can be less time-consuming, to cook from scratch.

The 'Oses'

Most sugars can be identified by the fact that they have an 'ose' at the end, glucose being the most obvious. So watch out for dextrose, maltose, sucrose, lactose, fructose.

Many of the foods that are marked as sugar-free are not actually sugar-free, as they could still contain carbohydrates or modified sugars. There is an assumption that anything that comes from fruit such as fructose is in fact healthy, but fructose will push up your blood-sugar level and cut out your ketone level at an alarmingly quick rate. When the ketone level is reduced, fat starts building up again. Also watch for things such as 'syrup': corn syrup, barley syrup, rice syrup and of course our old favorite golden syrup. These are all sugars, and should be avoided and included in the carbohydrate count. A possible exception to the sugars is 'xylose', xylitol. This sweetener is naturally occurring in our bodies and only has a glycemic index of 7; glucose has an index rating of 100. We do not recommend its continual use, but it can on occasion be used as a sweetener. Excessive amounts of xylose can operate as a laxative!

A bite of the apple

It is always assumed by people that eating fruit is the healthiest option available, but like all of these half-truths. fruit, for some, can have its downsides. When you are undertaking a ketogenic program, fruit is one of the things that has to be avoided. This is not stating that fruit is bad, but fruit has its own version of sugar, in the form of fructose (sometimes referred to as fruit sugar) that has its very sneaky metabolic pathway. Fructose — the fruit sugar — just like glucose has no place in a ketogenic diet. When faced with the choice on a ketogenic diet between fructose and glucose there is no choice, you cannot have either!

Fat is your friend because sugars are your enemy.

Fructose comes in various forms: some of them are modified. Possibly the worst form is high fructose corn syrup (HFCS). You will sometimes see this touted as a natural alternative to sugar. It's not. It's possibly the worst alternative to glucose that you could possibly consume.

Again, on a ketogenic diet HFCS has no place. Fructose can have a devastating effect on the cellular metabolism. In fact this effect can be more dramatic than glucose as fructose has the ability to skip some of the essential sugar-regulating biochemical functions.

Glucose — the sugar that most of you are aware of — is a 6-carbon aldehyde sugar. Fructose, which is often touted as the natural alternative, is a 6-carbon keto sugar. Insulin is required for normal cellular uptake of glucose. Fructose can enter the cells without the action of, or in the absence of, insulin. 3

This ability to enter cells without the intervention of insulin literally means that fructose can punch its way into the cells with no regulation; it has the ability to saturate the cellular function, overwhelming all the checks and balances.

The problem may arise with some people who have been eating incorrectly all their lives or are suffering from some form of chronic fatigue syndrome, reactive hypoglycemia or just basic sluggish metabolism, if there are problems with the mitochondria.

In this case fructose or glucose can be expected to generate a somewhat similar problem. At this point this is just a normal metabolic function. But high levels of glucose or high levels of fructose can cause the same metabolic disturbance —- fructose enters the cells more rapidly than glucose and insulin is not required as part of the regulatory process. 4

It is also metabolized more rapidly than glucose. This is due to the fact that the rate-limiting step, the reaction step in the chain of reactions of the glycolysis pathway that limits the speed of the pathway, is 'upstream' of the point at which fructose enters.

Or to put it more simply the fructose has sneaked by the regulation process that governs basic glucose and is pouring into the cells in the bloodstream with no form of regulation. There is no break or stop switch. The fructose train is out of control and heading for the end of the line.

Because of this rapid metabolism there can be an accumulation of the downstream products (glycolytic intermediates) such as fructose-1-phosphate. This occupies all available phosphate and leaves less cellular phosphate available for the formation of ATP (that amazing energy molecule upon which we run). This lack of ATP puts pressure on the cells for energy production.

As a result there can be increased glyogenolysis and this can then lead to a buildup of lactic acid and potentially fatal lactic acidosis. I must emphasize that fatal lactic acidosis is exceptionally rare but as you can see the act of consuming fructose is to drain the body of essential energy rather than adding to it. It does give an individual an immediate 'fructose hit' but this comes at a cost of a fundamental energy drain.

<u>The natural fat you eat whether saturated or not does not cause chronic disease, but the lack of it can.</u>

The bottom line is that on a ketogenic diet both forms of sugar are to be avoided. But the sugar contained in a piece of 95% chocolate (glucose) is far preferable to the sugar contained in a plum or a peach.

T. Kizhner, O. Shilovizki, M. Werman are the authors of a paper entitled 'Long-term fructose intake reduces oxidative defense and alters mitochondrial performance in mice'. Using electron microscopy, they found changes in mitochondrial morphology caused by the prolonged consumption of fructose and concluded that "These findings support the concern directed at the extensive use of fructose in the food industry." [5]

The authors of another paper conclude that "Whereas glucose favors overall growth kinetics, fructose enhances protein synthesis and appears to promote a more aggressive cancer phenotype. Fructose has become ubiquitous in our food supply, with the highest consumers being teens and young adults. Therefore, understanding the potential health consequences of fructose and its role in chronic disease development is of critical importance."[6]

Another scholarly article highlights the problems with pancreatic cancer. In this the authors found that "cancer cells can readily metabolize fructose to increase proliferation." They state that their findings "have major significance for cancer patients given dietary refined fructose consumption, and indicate that efforts to reduce refined fructose intake or inhibit fructose-mediated actions may disrupt cancer growth". [7]

Fat

We recommend fat, saturated fat, such as butter, lard, coconut oil and high fat cheese. We recommend extra-virgin olive oil. You need 75% of your calories from fat. Fats combined with protein will give more satiety than carbohydrates, so you need less to feel full. Fat is the fuel you will be burning on this diet, more satisfying and more efficient. The word fat in our language now has so many bad connotations from 'fat cats to fat hips'. In many the word triggers an instant fear reaction. A fear reaction can create cortisol release in the brain. It is an emotional response that kicks in the fear and anxiety, that fear and anxiety actually adds to your 'fat building' due to higher cortisol levels. The trick to remember is that fat burns fat and does not create it. Do not become a victim of 'ill informed choice', we can all remember that must have dress or pair of shoes that we simply had to have. We can also remember that sinking feeling we had when we wore them in public. To change how you view the consumption of fat just add this one little thought into your head when you eat it, 'healthy fat burning fat'. This will help short circuit the emotional fear that surrounds eating fat and of course add to your fat burning by helping dampen down the emotional cortisol release.

It is important to understand that in ketogenics we do not advise or recommend trans fats in your diet. Trans fats are often partly or wholly manufactured by chemical means; they are not processed or utilized by your metabolism in the same manner as naturally-occurring saturated fats. Think of them this way: animal fats like butter are a natural product, but trans fats are like a fatty 'play dough': you would not spread play dough on bread and expect it to be healthy. So take care and avoid the 'synthetic play dough' fats.

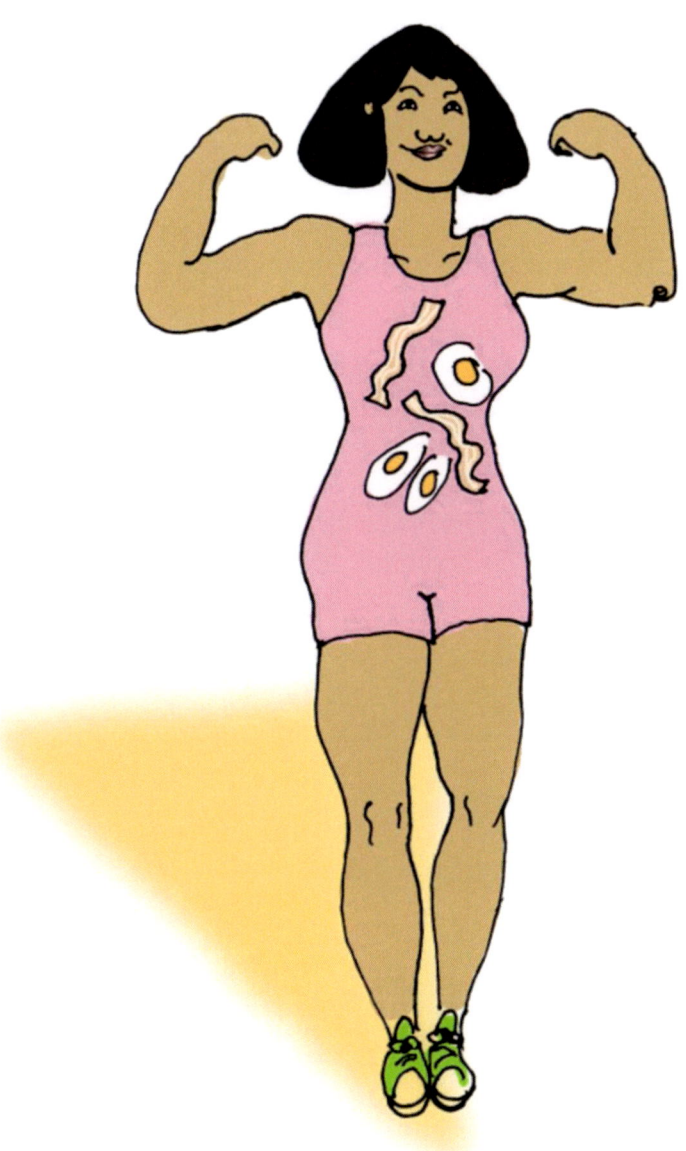

Menopause and Manopause

Many people reading this, especially women, tend to become a little alarmed over the quantity of fat required in a ketogenic diet. Hopefully our approach will not scare you away!

I will comment that if high-carbohydrate low-fat low-protein diets made you slim, energetic, menopause symptom-free and provided you with a sharp mind and flexible joints, why aren't you like that now?

If the low-fat high starch diets worked, there would only be one diet book on the shelves of a bookshop and that would be the end of the argument. They haven't worked because people have spent their lives going from one program to another and suffering the misery of having to watch and count what they eat all of the time; yet in spite of that the important fact is that as soon as they stopped, they gained weight and often they ended up in a worse condition than when they started.

Biochemically, there is no such thing as 'Manopause'. This is just the popular name used for andropause, but it does have remarkable similarities with menopause. You could say that both men and women at a certain age who have suffered from a high- sugar high-carbohydrate lifestyle begin to sink into a hormonal spiral that is remarkably similar.

What becomes obvious to most women as soon as they read the Wikipedia entry for menopause is that menopause is a natural process and that the symptoms commonly associated with menopause should not actually exist. 8 At menopause, when menstruation ceases, declining estrogen should be easily taken over by peripheral tissues of women's bodies. The adrenal glands produce androgen hormones, which convert into 75% the circulating estrogens in a woman's normal daily output, and into 100% of circulating estrogens after menopause. (Labrie 1991 Mol Cell Endocrinology) The reduction of estrogen hormone produced by the ovaries really should not create the large hormonal speed bump many books on menopause, and advertisements for "managing" menopause announce. Menopause is not and should not be a kind of impending doom scenario. Menopause is a clever female evolutionary strategy which actually helps women live long, productive, energetic lives by reducing the aging of other physiological systems. Mother nature actually knows what she is doing and when menopause works, as it is intended to do, it should represent a dream period of vitality in the female life cycle.

There is a lessening of hormonal function, but this lessening of hormonal function should not necessarily make you fat, tired, irritable, unable to concentrate and produce hot flushes/flashes. What is clear is that in its correct form menopause is no more than a transition from fertility to lack of fertility; it should not actually be a life-destroying spin of the coin.

In Manopause the situation is slightly more confusing as some of the experts are still arguing whether andropause actually exists at all. What is known is that men suffer the same erratic cortisol levels, poor insulin regulation and a diminishing of the essential male hormone testosterone.

These two sets of symptoms, apart from a few sets of hormonal precursors, produce identical symptoms in both men and women. It's just that in women they are more obvious than in men, and in men there has been a general acceptance that men get fat in middle age. Most of the symptoms associated with menopause and manopause are controllable and can be eliminated via a ketogenic diet.9

There is, however, one caveat to this problem. Some people have been subject for so long to a high-starch high-sugar diet that their ability to monitor blood sugar fluctuations and insulin production on a cellular level no longer exists. There is a percentage of people in the Western world who have become so damaged by sugar consumption in all its complex in various forms, they are unable to rectify the damage. Fortunately from experience we would say this is only one or 2% of the population. Patience and adjusting the ratio of fat to protein, and adding high fat snacks to your daily diet will help you overcome any blood sugar fluctuations until you are adapted to ketosis. Your health and how you feel is what is important. If you want to lose weight, you may need to consider if your ideal image of yourself is unrealistic and possibly unhealthy for you.

Understanding why the ketogenic diet works in Menopause and Manopause

It is now generally understood that we are designed to burn fat as our primary fuel source. It is also understood that under certain conditions our bodies will burn carbohydrates when the fat source of nutrition is exhausted.

The Western diet and many Eastern diets which are saturated in starches, carbohydrates, grains and sugars are actually fueling the secondary emergency system that we developed in Paleolithic times to run away from predators. The secondary system, or as we could define it the 'glucogenic system,' is governed by the adrenal hormone cortisol.

Do you remember the fight and flight principle from school biology lessons?
The function of cortisol is to raise blood sugar level under stress conditions; you could put it another way by saying the role of cortisol is to pour on a gallon of gasoline/petrol onto an already burning fire to create a rather spectacular burst of fire and heat, or in this case instant energy.

The key here being instant energy that is supposed to come and go very quickly but not persist. Long-term stress creates conditions in which the fire is always burning at its highest. It is important to understand that a body that is running on sugar will be recognized biochemically by the cells as one that is in a "stress condition" or under stress.

Being in a stress condition, all of the mechanisms that should function for a normal and gentle hormone and biochemical ebb and flow will be triggered into an alarm state. The body of a high-carbohydrate eater never actually rests.

Because the body of a high carbohydrate eater never rests, its physiological and biochemical systems are exhausted and wear out far more quickly.

A useful analogy would be getting a new car, filling the tank with rocket fuel and then driving it in low gear at high revs for its entire working life. A car subjected to that kind of abuse would wear out in a matter of years rather than decades. This is what happens to people, the high level of sugars literally grind your biochemical and physiological systems into old age and erratic function.

<u>A stable insulin level creates a stable hormonal function.</u>

With the dietary elevation of cortisol, there is a clear relationship with functional estrogenic levels. In its simplest explanation part of the role of the hormone estrogen is to allocate and steer glucose into the human brain for use as fuel. This is part of our emergency stress reaction process or to put it more simply the 'run like hell there's a tiger coming' syndrome.

In menopause it's already been noted that the hormone levels begin to drop, and with the reduction of these critical hormones the body and brain increasingly rely upon this emergency stress-based hormonal intervention. This doesn't matter when you are on a keto-adapted diet as you are actually running on your primary fuel source, fat generated ketones.

When you are keto-adapted your brain, muscles and other biochemical systems are no longer dependent upon sugar or this emergency switch to give you some semblance of energy and biochemical function.

In males as well as females, once your body is in a state of ketosis, there is an incredible hormonal advantage, that of stable insulin production. This may well help to both lose fat and regenerate muscle. In the weightlifting and muscle pumping world the main hormone they are concerned with is testosterone. It has been reported by many weightlifters, athletes and muscle builders that the ketogenic diet provides them with more usable energy and also elevates testosterone levels. An increased level of testosterone has multiple benefits throughout the male physiology, one of the most obvious being male sexual function. Who would have thought that long-term a pork chop could have actually the same effect as a little blue sildenafil citrate 'viagra' pill?

The commonly associated symptoms of low testosterone are:
Low libido
Erectile dysfunction
Fatigue
Reduced frequency of having a morning erection
Increased body fat, particularly around the waist
Reduced muscle mass and physical strength
Low motivation and self-confidence
Increased sweating
Sleep problems
Mood changes
Sedentary behavior

The commonly associated symptoms of Menopause are
Irregular periods
Vaginal dryness
Fatigue
Hot flashes
Night sweats
Sleep problems
Mood changes
Weight gain and slowed metabolism
Thinning hair and dry skin
Sedentary behavior

Common symptoms for type 2 diabetes
Excessive hunger for starches,sugars and or carbohydrates
Fatigue
Blurry vision
Sores or cuts that won't heal
Overweight
Sedentary behavior
High blood pressure
Excessive thirst
Frequent or increased urination, especially at night

As you can see there is considerable cross-over between the three lists. In practice all three conditions have been shown to respond well to a ketogenic diet.

The point of critical understanding is that if you are running on sugars only and your ability to produce insulin is compromised by long-term sugar, starch, carbohydrate consumption, your ability to shift glucose into the brain will fall.

Your brain, like all organs and glands, then registers its alarm of being starved of any form of energy and sends a hormonal message to your adrenal glands; this in turn stimulates the production of adrenal hormones epinephrine and norepinephrine, and as a result of this, cortisol levels will increase. Your brain has used the primitive message 'I am in danger' (a stress alarm message) and your body has responded with a kick of adrenaline to enable you to run away from danger (another stress alarm event). The effect of this is the heart rate goes up, we begin to sweat, get panicky and sometimes turn bright-red or in other words the commonly accepted symptoms of menopause. Some people with a very poorly adapted system will feel faint, have weak legs, feel nauseous and also have a sensation of feeling 'spaced out' and not quite able to think and function.

As a final thought ask yourself this how many of your friends who suffer many of these symptoms have actually been put on some form of tranquilizer or mood enhancing drug for what you can now clearly identify as an insulin/cortisol/adrenaline in balance?

As you can see from all of the above, ketogenic diets make sense on several levels for both immediate health and energy to long-term longevity and joyous health into old age. Every hormone works in a relative feedback mechanism with the other; the stabilizing effect the ketogenic diet has on a woman's endocrine system is remarkable. Think of all the times hormonal changes affect a woman's life. The ketogenic diet is beneficial each and every time hormone production changes or is destabilized in a woman's life.

ReGeneration-X Diet

You can kick-start your metabolism and generate lots of fat-burning energy by incorporating these recipes into your routine. Unlocking the self-healing potential of your body by eating a high-fat, low-carbohydrate diet with a moderate amount of protein is the most important part of the ReGeneration-X program. Having these recipes on hand will make it easier to plan your meals. After a few days you will get the hang of it, and automatically eat the right amount you need for your body. The easiest way to measure how much protein and fat is right for you is to eat 1 gram net protein for every kilogram of your desired weight. To calculate how much fat you need simply multiply the amount of protein in grams by three.

If you weigh 80kg, you need 80g of net fat protein (not lean protein), about 300g,or about 11oz of fat containing protein day. Measure the weight of your meat, chicken, or fish before you cook it. We calculate for net protein, as a good amount of water is lost when you cook it. The 300g of protein in volume could be divided into a two egg breakfast with bacon, 20g protein, a 100g portion of meat, fish, or chicken at lunch and dinner, as each 100g portion has about 24g of net protein.

On this diet the net fiber and carbohydrates come from your the vegetables. Eat as many vegetables as you like. They have very few carbohydrates. But this diet is mostly fat.
As 75% of your energy should come from the amount of fat you eat during the day, multiplying your daily net protein by three is the easiest way to calculate your daily fat need, or as in using the 80kg example, three times 80 equal 240, hence 240g of fat a day, from butter, coconut oil, or the fatty parts of meat. Remember, you do not count calories on this diet. Be aware that some protein sources have carbohydrate, such as mussels and dairy. The recipes below use moderate protein amounts and make up most of the fat requirement with pure fats, such as coconut oil or butter. It may be difficult to take in the amount of fat needed to go into ketosis initially. We have been brainwashed for over 50 years into avoiding fat. Melting 30g of fat into your favorite herbal tea is sometimes the easiest way to arrive at the best fat ratio. The great news is you don't need a calories counter, stick to grams and don't sweat the small stuff. Counting calories is a time wasting process, as your concern is fat, protein, and carbs. So donate your calorie manuals and battery operated calorie

counters to someone you do not like!

Keep in mind that some people find dairy increases their insulin level which can make ketosis difficult. If you find it hard to get into ketosis, eliminate dairy for a few days to see if it helps.

<u>Obesity is not caused by lack of will power, over-eating or lack of exercise. It's a starch excess and a lack of fat.</u>

Sometimes you may find the ketostix do not change color, signifying that you are not in ketosis. This may be due to several problems, such as insulin resistance, as in type 2 diabetes, hormonal changes due to menopause, or cortisol resistance for those leading a stressful life. It's a roll of the dice. Therefore we have designed the Jumpstart Keto Diet Plan, which you will find at the end of the recipes section.

The ratio of protein to fat in this diet will give you enough protein for your body's needs, but not too much for it to turn into glucose. This is a moderate protein diet designed to change your body's engine from glucose-burning to fat-burning. Your protein needs may vary according to the amount of physical activity you engage in.

We recommend you start with a simple menu, including items which are easy to find where you shop. The most important thing to remember is that this is a high-fat, moderate-protein diet. You can divide all the ingredients into three categories: fat, protein, and vegetables. You can increase the amount of fat, your new energy source, by cooking with it, and by adding it to drinks such as coffee, tea, herb tea, or even unsweetened cocoa made with water. It may take a few days to get used to not cutting off the fatty part of the meat, or skimping on the oil or butter when you cook. Just as your body has to become keto-adapted, you have to become used to this new/old way to cook. Fat is your friend.

How to know how much to eat

An easy way to calculate your macronutrient ratio on the diet is to take your desired weight, and calculate one net gram of protein for each kilogram. For example 100g in volume weight for a typical protein such as chicken or canned fish will give you about 25 net grams of protein. Multiply your daily requirement of net protein by three and you easily have the amount in grams of fat you need for the ketogenic diet. You will need more protein if you lead a very active life, both mentally and physically. Keep in mind however, that the older you are, the less protein you will need, and the more insulin resistant you are, the less protein you will need. If you are not in ketosis after 3 days on the diet, lower the protein and increase the amount of fat, or follow the Jumpstart Keto Diet Plan for 3 days.

Keep it simple

We have a huge variety available to us when we shop. Beginning this diet will be easier if you start off with some simple ingredients. Stick to the basics of eggs and bacon, or just eggs from the breakfast section. Choose a simple lunch and dinner, of a moderate serving of protein and a big salad, and you will find it easier.

Let's start with breakfast. What your mother told you was true, it is the most important meal of the day. Get the right mix of protein and fat first thing in the morning, and you start your body and mind off with enough fuel to last you until lunch, without sputtering for a break mid-morning.

Your body and mind are ready to go, first thing in the morning! The hormone Cortisol wakes you up, and your whole system expects you to go with it, so by eating a breakfast with enough protein and fat, you are giving it just what it needs to work with. However, if you are used to a small breakfast, start off with one egg instead of two, and whip your morning coffee or tea with a tablespoon of butter and coconut oil to give you the right amount of fat you need to give you the energy to start the day off right.

Buy:
coconut oil
heavy cream
lard
bacon
heavy cream
cheddar

mozzarella
parmesan
gorgonzola
eggs
canned sardines and mackerel
salmon filet
chicken thighs
pork chops
skirt steak
New York strip
rib-eye steak
avocados
all leafy green vegetables
green vegetables

Stop buying:
bread
crackers
cereal
granola
cookies
energy bars
pastry
pasta
rice
potatoes
corn

Drink:
water
herbal tea
morning coffee or tea

We're not talking about the International House of Pancakes-style breakfast with a stack of system-clogging carbohydrate flapjacks to make you want to lie down on the first couch you see, but eggs and bacon dressed up with creamy spinach, or asparagus spears.

Two eggs over easy with bacon isn't a complicated or time

consuming breakfast. You can make it in couple of minutes, or you can go to any diner and coffee shop to get them to make it for you.

We also recommend you start your day with a delicious cup of frothy butter and coconut oil coffee or tea. This will ensure you have plenty of energy in both body and mind well into lunchtime. It is also a good idea to drink decaffeinated butter coffee or tea in the afternoon to make it easier for you to get enough fat during the day. You will find this recipe in the fat buddies section.

Some important tips to remember on the ReGeneration-X diet:
Make sure each meal includes healthy saturated fat
Hard cheeses have equal amounts of fat and protein, so they are good for snacks
Nuts and nut butters have fat, carbohydrates, and protein, so limit these to stay below 20g of carbohydrate a day
Don't go too long between eating: snack on cured meats and drink decaffeinated butter tea or coffee in between meals
Stock the fridge with easy-to-prepare ReGeneration-X ingredients such as home-made dips, celery sticks and fennel
Keep hard-boiled eggs in the fridge
Never run out of butter, coconut oil, eggs, or cheese

The following recipes make two servings of each dish. The macronutrient values for each dish are equal to one serving.

Breakfast

Eggs and Bacon
Fat 35   Protein 20   Carb 1.5
4 eggs
8 slices bacon
2 cups/50g of arugula/rocket, washed with ends chopped off
2 tablespoons butter
salt and pepper to taste
2 eggs over easy with bacon with arugula/rocket.
In a pan cook bacon slices over medium heat, set aside.
Add 1 tablespoon of butter to the remaining bacon grease.
Crack two eggs into a pan, with fire still on medium.

When egg whites are firm, cover pan and turn off heat

I like to open yolks and let it flow over the arugula/rocket, so all the soft yolk gets eaten, but you can plate this however you wish.

Scrambled egg Florentine
Fat 36   Protein 12   Carb 2
Rinse fresh spinach three times, drain and towel dry, as spinach has lots of water in it, or simply use a bag of baby spinach.
4 eggs
2 cups/50g spinach
1/4 teaspoon nutmeg
1/4 cup heavy cream
2 tablespoon butter
salt and pepper to taste

Crack eggs into bowl.
Add nutmeg, salt and pepper, and heavy cream.
Beat with fork until well-combined.
Drop butter into medium-sized pan.
Add spinach, stir until cooked.
Add egg and cream mixture, toss lightly until eggs softly scrambled.

Pork sausage and fennel and beetroot hash
Fat 42   Protein 19   Carb 9
8 oz/225g sausage meat, chopped
1 medium fennel bulb, chopped into small cube-size pieces
1/2 a roasted beetroot
1 tablespoon chopped parsley
1/4 cup or 50g soaked walnuts, chopped

Cook sausage and fennel in a medium-sized pan.
When fennel starts to brown at the edges, add walnuts and pieces of beetroot.
Add parsley and salt and pepper to taste.

Asparagus provolone omelette
Fat 51   Protein 31   Carb 3
4 eggs

1/2 cup/100g provolone
2 teaspoons parsley
2 tablespoons heavy cream
salt and pepper to taste
8 asparagus spears, poached and chopped into bite-size pieces

Melt 2 oz butter in medium pan.
Turn fire to medium.
Beat eggs, cream, spices and parsley with a fork.
Pour egg mixture into pan.
When bottom of egg mixture is firm, add asparagus and cheese slices to half of egg mixture.
With spatula, gently lift uncovered part of omelette and fold it over asparagus and cheese.
Cook 2 minutes until cheese melts.
Cut in half, and serve, lifting pan and guiding omelette onto plate with spatula.

Smoked salmon blini with cream cheese
Fat 54   Protein 34   Carb   .39g
8oz/200g smoked salmon
2 tablespoons cream cheese
2 olive oil crepes/wraps
Fill each olive oil wrap with 4oz smoked salmon.
Add 1 tablespoon cream cheese.
Any fresh herb to your liking.

Calories counting is pointless, just cut the starches.

Lunch

Avocado stuffed with chicken salad
Fat 45   Protein 27   Carb 8
2 avocados
2 cups/200g cooked chicken breast, chopped and cubed
2 tablespoons mayonnaise
2 celery stalks, sliced finely
1/2 teaspoon paprika,
salt and pepper to taste

Mix ingredients above and spoon into avocado halves.

Fried eggplant, asparagus, and cheddar melt
Fat 55   Protein   12 Carb   12
1/2 medium firm eggplant, peeled and sliced lengthwise
8 asparagus spears, cut-off white bottom to light green part
4 oz cheddar cheese
1/4 cup/30g buckwheat flour for dredging eggplant
olive oil for frying eggplant

Poach asparagus spears in small amount of water.
Remove from water.
Sprinkle 2 teaspoons Himalayan salt onto eggplant.
Mix salt into eggplant gently with fingers.
Wait 15 minutes.
Rinse and drain.
Dry eggplant slices with paper towel.
Spread flour onto dinner plate, add salt to taste.
Cover bottom of large pan with olive oil.
Dredge each eggplant slice in buckwheat flour.
When oil is hot, place each slice into pan.
When one side is browned, turn over and brown other side.
Remove eggplant from pan and place onto plate covered with paper towels.

Heat oven to 350°/175°
Arrange four fried eggplant slices in flat baking dish.
Cover each eggplant slice with 2 asparagus spears lengthwise.
Add sliced cheddar pieces.
Cover with remaining eggplant slices.
Bake until cheese is melted.

Italian flag avocado salad
Fat 67   Protein 13   Carb 12
1 avocado
1 ripe tomato
1/2 cup/100g of fresh mozzarella cheese
romaine and arugula/rocket leaves washed

Slice avocado, tomato and cheese.
Spread salad and arugula/rocket on two plates.
Arrange avocado, tomato and mozzarella, alternating with each
ingredient to make the colors of the Italian flag.
Dress with oil and vinegar.

Canned mackerel or sardine salad
Fat 60   Protein 30   Carb   6
2 cans mackerel or sardines drained
100 grams or 2 cups mixed salad of wild radish, watercress,
arugula/rocket, and romaine
6 tablespoon of mayonnaise
1 tablespoon of capers chopped
4 small pickles chopped
6 walnuts
1 tablespoon parsley, chopped
1 fried egg, fried over easy.
1/4 teaspoon hot pepper
salt and pepper to taste

Cover two plates with salad.
Dress with oil and vinegar.
Mix all other ingredients in bowl.
Mix the above ingredients and divide onto plated salad.

Kale, spring onion and bacon frittata
Fat 46   Protein   12   Carb 7
2 cups/100g fresh kale, tough stalks removed
2 spring onions or half a red onion (spring onions and red onion are
much sweeter than onions)
4 slices chopped bacon
4 eggs
salt and pepper to taste
1/4 cup/50ml heavy cream (optional)
1 tablespoon chopped parsley
2 tablespoons, 30 gram butter

Beat eggs and cream by hand with fork.

Add salt and pepper.
Chop kale finely.
Sauté in olive oil until edges browned-kale gets sweeter when it is browned.
Add bacon and lower heat.
Stir well.
Pour egg mixture over kale and bacon.
Turn heat to medium and cook until egg starts to pull away from the edges, but top of eggs is still soft.
Put into pre-heated oven.
Cook until frittata firm, and center does not wobble.

Olive oil egg-wraps
Fat 40   Protein 6   Carb 4
2 eggs
2 tablespoon olive oil
1 tablespoon/15g butter
salt and pepper to taste

Beat eggs and oil well.
Butter small frying pan.
Pour in mixture.
Turn pan as for crepe.
Cover until firm on low heat.
Flip onto plate.
Makes 2 wraps
Fill with chopped smoked turkey and artichoke pesto
or cooked ground beef, sliced tomatoes and basil.

Mains

Meatloaf
Fat 67   Protein 39   Carb 6
Preheat oven to 325.
for meatloaf
1/2 lb./250g ground beef
1 egg
1 rye cracker crumbled
1/4 red onion chopped

1 tablespoon chopped parsley
1/2 cup heavy cream
salt and pepper to taste
1/2 cup tomato paste
1 tablespoon dijon mustard

Mix all ingredients except tomato paste and mustard in bowl.
Place meat in small loaf pan or medium oven proof frying pan.
Spread to cover bottom of pan.
Cook in oven for 40 minutes.
Mix tomato paste and mustard.
Spoon onto top of meat loaf, and cook for ten more minutes.
Remove from oven.
Allow to sit for 15 minutes.

Leftover meatloaf slices can be used for breakfast with eggs or lunch on a bed of salad the following day.

Oven barbecued spareribs
Fat 65   Protein   21   Carb 2

For sauce:
4 cups/400ml canned diced tomatoes
1/2 cup dijon mustard
1 cup/200ml apple cider vinegar
1/2 cup/100 soy sauce
Combine all ingredients in medium sauce pan and bring to a boil.
Cover and continue cooking on low heat for 1 hour.
1/2 cups soy sauce for rub
1 (2 to 3 lbs. rack pork ribs)

Then:

Rub ribs with salt, pepper and soy sauce and place in covered container in refrigerator overnight.
Pre-heat oven to 325°
Place rib on oven broiler and broil for 5 minutes, meat side up.
Roast ribs in oven for 2 1/2 hours, covering ribs with foil one hour into cooking to keep them moist.

Place on oven rack over a baking sheet covered with aluminum foil
After 2 hours using brush rub pork ribs with sauce, re-cover and finish cooking.

Fried fresh anchovies or sardines   with tartar sauce
Fat 40   Protein 25   Carb 10
1/2 lb./225g. fresh anchovies or sardine
1/4 cup/50g buckwheat flour
salt and pepper to taste
1 lemon
4 tablespoons olive oil
for tartar sauce
4 tablespoon mayonnaise
3 chopped pickles
1/4 teaspoon curry powder
1 tablespoon apple cider vinegar

Mix flour and spices together on a plate.
Dredge fish in flour mixture.
When oil is very hot add fish to pan one at a time.
Turn each fish separately when the bottom of the fish starts to brown.
Cook until both sides brown.
Remove from pan onto plate covered with paper towel.
Serve with fresh lemon slices.

Smoked ham casserole with artichokes
Fat 60   Protein 25   Carb 6
Pre-heat oven to 400°/200° degrees.

1/2 lb./225g smoked cooked boneless ham
1 cup/100gcherry tomatoes
1 cup/150g fresh peas
1 cup/150g fresh artichoke hearts, halved (you can also use thawed frozen hearts)
6 slices fatty bacon
1 tablespoon chopped basil
salt and pepper to taste

1/2 cup water

Add all ingredients to shallow 8/8 baking dish.
Put into oven and cook for 20 minutes, or until tomatoes become
soft and create a sauce.

Stir-fried shrimp and baby bok choy with red bell pepper
Fat 60   Protein 26   Carb 2
4-6 tb olive oil
1/2 lb./225 fresh or frozen shrimp
1/2 teaspoon garlic
1/2 red bell pepper, sliced into strips
2 cups/100g baby bok choy, chopped
1 tablespoon soy sauce
1 teaspoon apple cider vinegar
1/2 teaspoon Chinese 5 spice powder

Heat oil in medium pan.
Brown garlic and red pepper.
Add shrimp and bok choy.
Toss with spoon until cooked.
Add spices, vinegar, soy sauce.

Yankee pot roast
Fat 60   Protein   21   Carb 2
1/2 lb./225g boneless chuck roast
6 tablespoon butter
1/3 cup /100mlapple cider vinegar
2 tablespoon soy sauce
5 cups/1 liter water
2 teaspoons black pepper
Add meat and butter to pan large enough to cover meat with lid.
Brown meat on both sides with butter.
Add remaining ingredients.
Cook on high heat for 30 minutes.
Simmer for 3 hours on low heat.
Make sure there is always liquid in bottom of pan.
If not add more water.

Pot roast zucchini/courgette hash
Fat 47   Protein 24   Carb 4
Left over pot roast
1/2/100ml cup tomato sauce
2 eggs
1 zucchini/courgette, roughly chopped
1/4 cup whole milk
salt and pepper to taste

Chop and shred left over pot roast
Drizzle olive oil on bottom of medium pan
Add meat.
Add tomato sauce.
Heat to simmering.
Add 2 beaten eggs and milk.
Stir mixture until eggs just cooked.
Salt and pepper to taste.

Sides

Mustard greens with provolone cheese
Fat 40   Protein   12Carb 2
2 cups mustard greens
1/2 cup/100g provolone
1/4 cup/50ml water
2 tablespoon olive oil
salt and pepper to taste

Add 2 tablespoon olive oil to medium pan.
Add mustard greens.
When greens are sautéed add and 1/4 cup water.
Cover for 5 minutes.
Uncover and continue cooking until most of the water has been absorbed.
Add chopped provolone cheese.
Stir on low fire to melt cheese with greens.

Cabbage carrot coleslaw

Fat 45   Protein 4   Carb 10
1/2 cabbage
1 carrot
4 tablespoon mayonnaise
2 tablespoon olive oil
1 tablespoon apple cider vinegar
1/2 teaspoon fresh ground black pepper
blend mayonnaise, olive oil, vinegar and pepper into a medium
mixing bowl
slice cabbage thin and put into bowl
grate carrot over cabbage
add parsley
mix well with large spoon

Sautéed kale with garlic and walnuts
Fat 60   Protein 7   Carb 6
4 tablespoon butter or olive oil
1/2 cup walnuts
2 cups /100gchopped kale
1 clove garlic

Arugula/Rocket and beet salad with shavings of parmesan with balsamic vinegar
Fat 50   Protein 35   Carb 8
2 cups of arugula/rocket
1/2 cup/50g roasted beet
1/2 cup/50g parmesan shavings
1/4 cup/50g pancetta cubes
1teaspoons balsamic vinegar
2 tablespoon olive oil

Sautéed fennel slices with cream cheese, coriander and balsamic vinegar
Fat 35   Protein 1   Carb 5
1 fennel bulb
1 tablespoon olive oil
1/2 cup/100g cream cheese
1 teaspoon balsamic vinegar
1/4 teaspoon ground coriander

Slice fennel lengthwise.
Sauté in hot oil briefly until brown edges of both sides brown.
Arrange slices on plates.
Dollop cream cheese onto hot fennel.
Add a dash of balsamic vinegar
and a sprinkle of coriander.

Zucchini/Courgette noodles in peanut sesame sauce
Fat 40   Protein 8   Carb 8
1 zucchini/courgette cut into medium slices, then cut each slice into
lengthwise to make noodle shape
2 teaspoon fresh ginger
1/2 teaspoon garlic
2 tablespoons peanut butter
4 tablespoons soy sauce
1 teaspoon apple cider vinegar
1 tablespoon water
1 tablespoon sesame oil
2 cups bean sprouts

Brown garlic and ginger in sesame oil.
Add all ingredients except for zucchini/courgette.
Mix well on low heat.
Heat 1 tablespoon sesame oil until hot.
Add zucchini/courgette strips, toss for 5 seconds.
Then add zucchini/courgette to sauce and stir gently.

Steamed cauliflower salad with salami and mustard dressing
Fat 50   Protein 18   Carb 3
2 cups steamed cauliflower
1/2 cup salami slices
4 tablespoons olive oil
1 tablespoon whole grain Dijon mustard
1 tablespoon mayonnaise
fresh ground pepper

Prepare the dressing with the olive oil, mustard and mayonnaise.
Put the cauliflower heads into a mixing bowl.
Add the dressing and toss.

Distribute onto 2 plates and top with salami slices and freshly ground black pepper

Fried green tomato mozzarella sandwiches
Fat 31   Protein 11   Carb 10
2 green tomatoes
4 oz/100g fresh mozzarella
1/4 cup/50g buckwheat flour
1/4 cup/50g corn meal
1/2 teaspoon salt
1/8 teaspoon ground hot pepper

Cut tomatoes into 1/2 inch slices.
Slice mozzarella into slices.
Heat medium pan.
Cover with olive oil.
Make sandwiches with tomato slices with mozzarella in between.
Holding sandwiches together dredge into flour mixture.
With spatula place each sandwich in hot oil.
When bottom tomato starts to brown at edges and cheese starts to melt, turn sandwich over.
Cook until cheese entirely melted.
Remove from pan with spatula onto plates.

Dips for celery sticks

Artichoke heart dip
Fat 52   Protein 7   Carb 8
1 8oz/200g package of frozen artichoke hearts (thawed)
1/2 cup/50g parsley leaves
1/2 cup/50g walnuts
1 clove garlic
1/2 cup/50g parmesan crumbled into small pieces
salt and pepper to taste
1/2 cup olive oil

Put all ingredients except olive oil in food processor.
Run until all ingredients are a chunky mix.

Add olive oil.
Keep in refrigerator in covered container for up to 4 days.

Cauliflower dip
Fat 55   Protein 9   Carb 2
2 cups steamed cauliflower florets
1/2 c /100g feta cheese
1/2 cup watercress, chopped
1 garlic clove
Place all ingredients in food processor.
Run until ingredients blended.
2 tablespoon olive oil
salt and pepper to taste
keeps in refrigerator in covered container for up to 4 days

*Eggplant tahini di*p
Fat 60   Protein 3   Carb 7
1 medium eggplant, peeled and chopped into cubes
1/2 cup/200ml olive oil
2 tablespoons tahini sauce
juice of 1 medium lemon
1 teaspoon coriander powder
salt and pepper to taste

Sprinkle eggplant with salt and let sit for 15 minutes.
Drain and rinse, squeezing water out of eggplant.
Put into hot large pan with 1/2 cup olive oil.
Sauté until eggplant soft and browned.
Turn off heat.
Mash eggplant with back of wooden spoon.
Add remaining ingredients and stir until blended.
Keep in refrigerator in covered container for up to 4 days.

Parsley dip
Fat 55   Protein 6   Carb 2
1 rye cracker
1/4 cup red wine vinegar
1 cup/100g parsley
1 clove garlic

1 pinch salt
1/2 cup walnuts
3 tablespoon capers
2 hardboiled eggs
4 pitted black olives
1 cup olive oil
Place ingredients in food processor.
Run until a smooth paste is made.
Keep in refrigerator in covered container for up to 4 days.

Fat buddies

Coffee with butter and coconut oil
1 regular cup of coffee or American coffee
2 tablespoon butter
1 tablespoon coconut oil
a pinch of cinnamon and bittersweet raw chocolate powder
(optional)
Blend until frothy.

Green tea with coconut oil
1 cup of tea with 2 tablespoons of coconut oil
Blend until frothy.

Verbena tea with coconut oil
1 cup of tea with 2 tablespoons of coconut oil
Blend until frothy.

Creamy chocolate coconut peanut butter (the easy fat snack)
1 jar coconut puree (215g or 15 oz jar is common)
2 tb coconut oil
2 tb creamy peanut butter
2 teaspoon raw cocoa powder

Heat jar of coconut puree in sauce pan.
Add enough water to immerse jar halfway.
Cover pan,
Over medium fire bring to boil for 10 minutes.
Remove jar with tongs.

Cool five minutes.
Add remaining ingredients,
Cool completely.

Simple desserts

When we think about the 'forbidden' foods we have been brainwashed to think of fatty foods as negative poor performers that damage one's health. We have told you that on the ReGeneration-X diet you can eat all the bacon, cream, and full-fat cream you have always wanted. We crave fat because we need it. If we think about the desserts that were popular in the 1950s, pre-Ancel Keys, his flawed Seven Countries Study of 1958, and the subsequent cholesterol scare (I have inherited a beautiful copy of Better Homes and Garden New Cookbook from 1953), they are full of full-fat chiffon berry pies, buttery blueberry, chocolate and sauces, creamy buttery fillings for meringues of all flavors from vanilla, to chocolate, to raspberry, to coconut. Fat, fat, fat, egg, egg, egg, butter, butter, butter. The only problem with these wonderful recipes is the sugar which is the 'negative impact' culprit in poor health.

After 1958, it was basically "let them eat cake". Layer cakes, cupcakes, and muffins with a little creamy frosting on top, or worse, just a sugary glaze. While a cake once in a while is fine on the ReGeneration-X diet, you can enjoy buttery, creamy desserts more of the time, without spiking your insulin levels and undoing all the hard work you have done to stabilize your insulin levels and lower your blood sugar. Once you are keto-adapted simply adding berries, unsweetened chocolate powder, and coconut flakes will give enough sweetness to these creamy desserts. We recommend first trying these recipes without any sweetener.

Inulin based sweeteners are natural starches which can be used to sweeten your desserts. They are made out of starches such as chicory root and jerusalem artichokes. Studies show they have a beneficial effect on blood sugar, but that being said they are still a starch, a should be used in moderation. We do not recommend Xylitol, Stevia and Erythritol, which are all sugar alcohol sweeteners and are hundreds of times sweeter-tasting than sugar. Your brain may confuse this burst of sweetness with the real thing, and consequently raise your insulin levels out of expectation. Do not confuse these sugar analogs with artificial sweeteners such as Aspartame and Sucralose.

All of the ingredients in these recipes are part of the ReGeneration-X Diet. The raw chocolate chips are loaded with healthy cocoa fat. Coconut flakes are satisfyingly crunchy and have almost zero carbs. Egg yolks are loaded with fat and egg whites are pure protein. Not a carbohydrate in sight.

<u>Eat until you are full, not stuffed. If you are hungry, increase fat.</u>

These are classic 1950s dessert recipes. Pierre Mattia remembers eating chocolate and lemon cream sandwiched between two fresh meringues from the dairy merchant in his home town of Sanremo. His father used to make fresh hot zabaglione (hold the Marsala) for him, his brother and his sister as a full-fat treat on cold winter mornings before school.

Zabaglione

6 egg yolks
Marsala (Optional)
Whip the yolks and sugar together with a whisk or an electric mixer (my preference) in a double boiler.
You can also put a smaller pot into a bigger pot filled with gently simmering water.
Marsala is a fortified wine, so it is low carb.
You can use a tablespoon or two of Marsala,
Continue to beat the mixture about 10 minutes, until it swells and forms soft, almost elastic, mounds. Pour into dessert cups and serve warm.

Meringues
3 egg whites
1 teaspoon vanilla extract
1/4 teaspoon cream of tartar

Separate egg whites from yolks at room temperature
(use the yolks for making zabaglione)
Add cream of tartar, vanilla, and a dash of salt.
Beat until soft peaks form.
Cover baking sheet with ungreased oven paper.
Dollop beaten egg white with a tablespoon onto paper.
Bake at 275°/125° for 1 hour.
Turn oven off and let meringues dry in oven with door closed for
two hours.
Take two, and use either a butter frosting or creamy filling for the
Italian meringue sandwich.

Egg custard sauce
In heavy saucepan mix 4 beaten egg yolks.
Add dash of salt.
Stir in 2 cups of full fat cream.
Cook over low heat, stirring constantly.
Remove from heat; cool pan at once in cold water.
Stir two minutes.
Add vanilla or raw, unsweetened chocolate powder to taste.

Blueberry sauce
In a heavy saucepan, over a very low fire,
melt 1/4 cup/50g butter.
Add dash of salt.
Add 2 cups/500g fresh blueberries.
Bring to light boil.
Remove from heat.
Stir in 3 tablespoons lemon juice.

Buttery frosting
You can flavor this frosting any way you like with
chocolate powder, vanilla extract, cinnamon, instant coffee, as long as
flavoring is a sugar-free extract, so as not to interfere with the
frosting's creamy consistency.

1/2 cup/100g butter
1/4 cup/50ml heavy cream
Cream butter.

Add enough cream to make frosting spreadable.
For a creamier texture beat in 1 egg and
reduce the amount of heavy cream by half.

Whipped cream sauce
2 cups/500ml heavy whipping cream
Beat heavy whipping cream until foamy in texture.
Take care not to over beat or you will make butter.
Flavor with berry sauce, or
raw chocolate chips, or coconut flakes, and cinnamon,
Whatever suits you!

Berry parfait
10 oz/200g package of frozen berries (raspberry, blueberry,
blackberry) thawed
2 teaspoons lemon juice
1 cup/220 ml heavy whipping cream
Heat thawed berries and juice on low fire.
Stir in sweetener and lemon juice.
Heat until mixture thickens slightly.
Pour into 2 parfait cups.
Cover with sweetened whipped cream.

Chocolate soufflé
1/3 cup/80ml heavy cream
3 oz/85g of cream cheese
3 egg yolks
3 egg whites

Preheat oven to 300°/175°

In heavy saucepan, blend cream and cheese over very low heat;
add chocolate chips; cook and stir to melt; cool.
Beat egg yolks with dash of salt till thick and lemon-colored (5
minutes).
Slowly blend in cooled chocolate.
Beat whites to soft peaks; gradually add sugar, beating into stiff
peaks.
Gently fold small amount of whites into chocolate mixture.

Then fold chocolate mixture into beaten egg whites in small batches.
Pour mixture into ungreased 1quart soufflé dish.
Bake at 300° for 50 minutes or sharp knife inserted halfway between center and edge of
soufflé comes out clean.
Remove soufflé gently from oven and place gently onto counter.
Serve with custard sauce or with zabaglione.

Jumpstart Keto Diet Plan

Eat this way for up to five days.

Breakfast
2 eggs cooked in 2 tb/30g butter
or
1 egg with 30 to 50g fatty bacon
sea salt to taste

Coffee or tea with butter and coconut oil

Lunch
4oz/100g fish/meat/fowl
2 cup/50g veg/salad
2tb/30g butter/coconut oil for cooking or dressing
sea salt to taste

Snack
handful of soaked nuts or 1oz/30g hard cheese

Dinner
4oz/100g fish/meat/fowl
2 cup/50g veg/salad
2tb/30g butter/coconut oil for cooking or dressing
sea salt to taste

Drink 2 liters of water a day.
Make sure you salt your food with good quality sea salt.
Carbohydrates make you retain salt. You need more in ketosis.
If you are hungry…eat spoonfuls of coconut oil or spoonfuls of

creamy chocolate coconut peanut butter from the fat buddies section and double amount of butter/coconut oil for cooking your dishes.

Vegan Recipes

There are many choices for today's ketogenic vegan chef. There is a strong vegan tradition in China. Vegan restaurants in China have always catered to vegan and non-vegan tastes, offering a dizzying variety of flavors which are often impossible to distinguish from meat and fish. I once traveled to Guandong with some of my students, and purposely did not tell a staunch meat-eater in my group that the barbequed pork he so enjoyed was made out of seitan until after we had finished our delicious meal. He still does not believe that he was in a vegan restaurant. The vegan diet does not have to be a carbohydrate laden, blood sugar rollercoaster. Coconut oil, a healthy saturated fat, is readily available in most health food stores. Good quality organic tofu and seitan is rich in vegetable protein and low in carbohydrates. Many of the vegan cheeses you find also include coconut oil and coconut flour as ingredients, making them ideal for the ketogenic vegan chef. Remember to you check the amount of carbohydrate indicated on the label. If you maintain the fat to protein ratio necessary to maintain ketosis, you will be fat-adapted and do well on a ketogenic vegan diet. I recommend supplementing with vitamin B12 if you are following the ketogenic vegan diet.

Scrambled Tofu Florentine
Fat 36   Protein 12   Carb 2
Rinse fresh spinach three times, drain and towel dry, as spinach has lots of water in it, or simply use a bag of baby spinach.
225g/8 oz tofu
2 cups/50g spinach
1/4 teaspoon nutmeg
1/4 cup coconut milk
2 tablespoon coconut oil
salt and pepper to taste

crumble tofu in a bowl
Add nutmeg, salt and pepper, and coconut cream.

Beat with fork until well-combined.
Drop oil into medium-sized pan.
Add spinach, stir until cooked.
Add tofu and cream mixture, toss lightly until softly scrambled.

Seitan and fennel and beetroot hash
Fat 42   Protein 19   Carb 9
8 oz/225g seitan, chopped
1 medium fennel bulb, chopped into small cube-size pieces
1/2 a roasted beetroot
1 tablespoon chopped parsley
1/4 cup or 50g soaked walnuts, chopped
olive oil

Cook seitan and fennel in a medium-sized pan.
When fennel starts to brown at the edges, add walnuts and pieces of beetroot.
Add parsley and salt and pepper to taste.

Nut and see muesli
Fat 50   Protein 19   Carb 6
4 oz/50g chia seeds
4 oz/50g almonds or walnuts
4 oz/50g coconut milk
4 oz/50g mixed berries
1 cup water
2 tb/30g coconut oil

Soak all nuts and seeds overnight in 1 cup of water.
Add all ingredients to sauce pan and heat over low fire, adding water if necessary for creaminess.
Serve.

Lunch

Avocado stuffed with smoked tofu salad
Fat 45   Protein 27   Carb 8
2 avocados
2 cups/200g smoked tofu, chopped and cubed
2 tablespoons eggless mayonnaise
2 celery stalks, sliced finely
10 small black olives, pitted and chopped
1/2 teaspoon paprika,
salt and pepper to taste

Mix ingredients above and spoon into avocado halves.

Fried eggplant, asparagus, and dairy-free cheddar melt
Fat 55   Protein   12 Carb   12
1/2 medium firm eggplant, peeled and sliced lengthwise
8 asparagus spears, cut-off white bottom to light green part
4 oz dairy-free cheddar cheese
1/4 cup/30g buckwheat flour for dredging eggplant
olive oil for frying eggplant

Poach asparagus spears in small amount of water.
Remove from water.
Sprinkle 2 teaspoons Himalayan salt onto eggplant.
Mix salt into eggplant gently with fingers.
Wait 15 minutes.
Rinse and drain.
Dry eggplant slices with paper towel.
Spread flour onto dinner plate, add salt to taste.
Cover bottom of large pan with olive oil.
Dredge each eggplant slice in buckwheat flour.
When oil is hot, place each slice into pan.
When one side is browned, turn over and brown other side.
Remove eggplant from pan and place onto plate covered with paper towels.

Heat oven to 350°/175°
Arrange four fried eggplant slices in flat baking dish.

Cover each eggplant slice with 2 asparagus spears lengthwise.
Add sliced cheddar pieces.
Cover with remaining eggplant slices.
Bake until dairy-free cheese is melted.

Italian flag avocado salad
Fat 67   Protein 13   Carb 12
1 avocado
1 ripe tomato
1/2 cup/100g of dairy-free mozzarella cheese
Romaine and arugula/rocket leaves washed

Slice avocado, tomato and cheese.
Spread salad and arugula/rocket on two plates.
Arrange avocado, tomato and mozzarella, alternating with each
ingredient to make the colors of the Italian flag.
Dress with oil and vinegar.

Seitan Viennese Wurstel salad
Fat 60   Protein 30   Carb   6
200g or 1 cup chopped Seitan Viennese Wurstel
100 grams or 2 cups mixed salad of wild radish, watercress,
arugula/rocket, and romaine
6 tablespoon of eggless mayonnaise
1 tablespoon of capers chopped
4 small pickles chopped
6 walnuts
1 tablespoon parsley, chopped
1/4 teaspoon hot pepper
salt and pepper to taste

Cover two plates with salad.
Dress with oil and vinegar.
Mix all other ingredients in bowl.
Mix the above ingredients and divide onto plated salad.

Kale, spring onion and seitan frittata
Fat 46   Protein   12   Carb 7

2 cups/100g fresh kale, tough stalks removed
2 spring onions or half a red onion (spring onions and red onion are much sweeter than onions)
125g or ½ cup soft tofu
salt and pepper to taste
1/4 cup/50ml coconut cream (optional)
1 tablespoon chopped parsley
2 tablespoons, 30 gram olive oil

Mix silken tofu and coconut cream by hand with fork.
Add salt and pepper.
Chop kale finely.
Sauté in olive oil until edges browned-kale gets sweeter when it is browned.
Stir well.
Pour tofu mixture over kale and seitan bacon.
Turn heat to medium and cook until tofu browns at the edges.
Put into pre-heated oven.
Cook until frittata firm, and center does not wobble.

Mains

Vegan lasagne

Preheat oven to 400°/200°
200g /1 cup seitan
200g /1 cup lightly cooked and still firm egg-free lasagna pasta
100g/1/2 cup soft or silken Tofu
200g/4 cups fresh spinach
100g/1 cup mushrooms
Parsley
Garlic
Olive oil

Cook spinach in skillet with olive oil and garlic, salt and pepper to taste, set aside
Cook mushrooms with olive oil, garlic and chopped parsley, salt and pepper to taste, set aside

In large skillet, preferably cast iron, well oiled with olive oil, place one layer of pasta.
to cover the bottom.
Cover with cooked spinach.
Add mushrooms.
Add thin slices of seitan to cover
Add slices of fresh tofu, or spoonfuls of creamy tofu to cover
Add one more layer of pasta
Repeat all of the above in the same order
Add one more layer of pasta to the second toppings
Add slices of fresh tofu or spoonfuls of silken tofu
Sprinkle with chopped parsley, fresh ground pepper and salt.
Cook in oven for 30 minutes.

Leftover lasagne slices can be used for breakfast or lunch on a bed of salad the following day.

Oven barbecued Seitan Ribs
Fat 65   Protein   21   Carb 2

For sauce:
4 cups/400ml canned diced tomatoes
1/2 cup dijon mustard
1 cup/200ml apple cider vinegar
1/2 cup/100 soy sauce
Combine all ingredients in medium sauce pan and bring to a boil.
Cover and continue cooking on low heat for 1 hour.
1/2 cups soy sauce for rub
500g/1 lb seitan

Then:

Marinate seitan with salt, pepper and soy sauce and place in covered container in refrigerator overnight.
Pre-heat oven to 325°/175°
Remove seitan from marinade.
Place seitan on oven broiler and broil for 5 minutes on each side.
Cover with sauce and roast seitan in oven 15 min. hour, covering it

with foil keep it moist.
Finish cooking for until sauce becomes crusty on surface.

Smoked Tofu casserole with artichokes
Fat 60   Protein 25   Carb 6
Pre-heat oven to 400°/200° degrees.

1/2 lb./225g smoked cooked boneless ham
1 cup/100g cherry tomatoes
1 cup/150g fresh peas
1 cup/150g fresh artichoke hearts, halved (you can also use thawed frozen hearts)
1 tablespoon chopped basil
salt and pepper to taste
1/2 cup water

Add all ingredients to shallow 8/8 baking dish.
Put into oven and cook for 20 minutes, or until tomatoes become soft and create a sauce.

Stir-fried vegetarian burger and baby bok choy with red bell pepper
Fat 60   Protein 26   Carb 2
4-6 tb olive oil
1/2 lb./225 vegetarian burger cut lengthwise
1/2 teaspoon garlic
1/2 red bell pepper, sliced into strips
2 cups/100g baby bok choy, chopped
1 tablespoon soy sauce
1 teaspoon apple cider vinegar
1/2 teaspoon Chinese 5 spice powder

Heat oil in medium pan.
Brown garlic and red pepper.
Add burger slices and bok choy.
Toss with spoon until cooked.
Add spices, vinegar, soy sauce.

Fried seitan paddies
Fat 50   Protein 23   Carb 15
150g/6 oz of seitan, sliced in half so they are cut into 2 even layers
25g/2 tb cornmeal
25/2 tb flour
50ml/1/4 cup coconut milk
heat cast-iron skillet with peanut oil until hot.
Mix flours with salt and pepper to taste.
Dip seitan slices in coconut milk.
Dredge slices in flour mixture.
Repeat.
Fry slices until golden brown.
Serve with barbeque sauce heated with 4 tb coconut oil

Sides

Mustard greens with dairy-free provolone cheese
Fat 40   Protein 12   Carb 2
2 cups mustard greens
1/2 cup/100g provolone
1/4 cup/50ml water
2 tablespoon olive oil
salt and pepper to taste

Add 2 tablespoon olive oil to medium pan.
Add mustard greens.
When greens are sautéed add and 1/4 cup water.
Cover for 5 minutes.
Uncover and continue cooking until most of the water has been absorbed.
Add chopped dairy-free provolone cheese.
Stir on low fire to melt cheese with greens.

Cabbage carrot coleslaw
Fat 45   Protein 4   Carb 10
1/2 cabbage
1 carrot
4 tablespoon egg-free mayonnaise

2 tablespoon olive oil
1 tablespoon apple cider vinegar
1/2 teaspoon fresh ground black pepper
blend mayonnaise, olive oil, vinegar and pepper into a medium
mixing bowl
slice cabbage thin and put into bowl
grate carrot over cabbage
add parsley
mix well with large spoon

Sautéed kale with garlic and walnuts
Fat 60   Protein 7   Carb 6
4 tablespoon butter or olive oil
1/2 cup walnuts
2 cups /100gchopped kale
1 clove garlic

*Arugula/Rocket and beet salad with shavings of dairy-free feta cheese with
balsamic vinegar*
Fat 50   Protein 35   Carb 8
2 cups of arugula/rocket
1/2 cup/50g roasted beet
1/2 cup/50g dairy free feta cheese
1/4 cup/50g smoked tofu cubes
1teaspoons balsamic vinegar
2 tablespoon olive oil

Sautéed fennel slices with cream cheese, coriander and balsamic vinegar
Fat 35   Protein 1   Carb 5
1 fennel bulb
1 tablespoon olive oil
1/2 cup/100g soy yoghurt cheese
1 teaspoon balsamic vinegar
1/4 teaspoon ground coriander

Slice fennel lengthwise.
Sauté in hot oil briefly until brown edges of both sides brown.
Arrange slices on plates.
Dollop cream cheese onto hot fennel.

Add a dash of balsamic vinegar
and a sprinkle of coriander.

Zucchini/Courgette noodles in peanut sesame sauce
Fat 40   Protein 8   Carb 8
1 zucchini/courgette cut into medium slices, then cut each slice into
lengthwise to make noodle shape
2 teaspoon fresh ginger
1/2 teaspoon garlic
2 tablespoons peanut butter
4 tablespoons soy sauce
1 teaspoon apple cider vinegar
1 tablespoon water
1 tablespoon sesame oil
2 cups bean sprouts

Brown garlic and ginger in sesame oil.
Add all ingredients except for zucchini/courgette.
Mix well on low heat.
Heat 1 tablespoon sesame oil until hot.
Add zucchini/courgette strips, toss for 5 seconds.
Then add zucchini/courgette to sauce and stir gently.

Steamed cauliflower salad with vegan salami and mustard dressing
Fat 50   Protein 18   Carb 3
2 cups steamed cauliflower
1/2 cup vegan salami slices
4 tablespoons olive oil
1 tablespoon whole grain dijon mustard
1 tablespoon mayonnaise
fresh ground pepper

Prepare the dressing with the olive oil, mustard and mayonnaise.
Put the cauliflower heads into a mixing bowl.
Add the dressing and toss.

Distribute onto 2 plates and top with salami slices and freshly ground
black pepper

Fried green tomato and tofu sandwiches
Fat 31   Protein 11   Carb 10
2 green tomatoes
4 oz/100g tofu cheese
1/4 cup/50g buckwheat flour
1/4 cup/50g corn meal
1/2 teaspoon salt
1/8 teaspoon ground hot pepper

Cut tomatoes into 1/2 inch slices.
Slice tofu into slices.
Heat medium pan.
Cover with olive oil.
Make sandwiches with tomato slices with tofu in between.
Holding sandwiches together dredge into flour mixture.
With spatula place each sandwich in hot oil.
When bottom tomato starts to brown at edges and cheese starts to melt, turn sandwich over.
Cook golden brown.
Remove from pan with spatula onto plates.

Dips for celery sticks

Artichoke heart dip
Fat 52   Protein 7   Carb 8
1 8oz/200g package of frozen artichoke hearts (thawed)
1/2 cup/50g parsley parsley leaves
1/2 cup/50g walnuts
1 clove garlic
1/2 cup/50g soy yoghurt crumbled into small pieces
salt and pepper to taste
1/2 cup olive oil

Put all ingredients except olive oil in food processor.
Run until all ingredients are a chunky mix.
Add olive oil.
Keep in refrigerator in covered container for up to 4 days.

Cauliflower dip
Fat 55   Protein 9   Carb 2
2 cups steamed cauliflower florets
1/2 c /100g coconut cream
1/2 cup watercress, chopped
1 garlic clove
Place all ingredients in food processor.
Run until ingredients blended.
2 tablespoon olive oil
salt and pepper to taste
keeps in refrigerator in covered container for up to 4 days

*Eggplant tahini di*p
Fat 60   Protein 3   Carb 7
1 medium eggplant, peeled and chopped into cubes
1/2 cup/200ml olive oil
2 tablespoons tahini sauce
juice of 1 medium lemon
1 teaspoon coriander powder
salt and pepper to taste

Sprinkle eggplant with salt and let sit for 15 minutes.
Drain and rinse, squeezing water out of eggplant.
Put into hot large pan with 1/2 cup olive oil.
Sauté until eggplant soft and browned.
Turn off heat.
Mash eggplant with back of wooden spoon.
Add remaining ingredients and stir until blended.
Keep in refrigerator in covered container for up to 4 days.

Parsley dip
Fat 55   Protein 6   Carb 2
1 rye cracker
1/4 cup red wine vinegar
1 cup/100g parsley
1 clove garlic
1 pinch salt
1/2 cup walnuts
3 tablespoon capers

50 g/1/4 cup silken tofu
4 pitted black olives
1 cup olive oil
Place ingredients in food processor.
Run until a smooth paste is made.
Keep in refrigerator in covered container for up to 4 days.

Fat buddies
Coffee with butter and coconut oil
1 regular cup of coffee or American coffee
2 tablespoon coconut cream
1 tablespoon coconut oil
a pinch of cinnamon and bittersweet raw chocolate powder
(optional)
Blend until frothy.

Green tea with coconut oil
1 cup of tea with 2 tablespoons of coconut oil
Blend until frothy.

Verbena tea with coconut oil
1 cup of tea with 2 tablespoons of coconut oil
Blend until frothy.

Creamy chocolate coconut peanut butter (the easy fat snack)
1 jar coconut puree (215g or 15 oz jar is common)
2 tb coconut oil
2 tb creamy peanut butter
2 teaspoon raw cocoa powder

Heat jar of coconut puree in sauce pan.
Add enough water to immerse jar halfway.
Cover pan,
Over medium fire bring to boil for 10 minutes.
Remove jar with tongs.
Cool five minutes.
Add remaining ingredients,
Cool completely

Simple Vegan desserts

Creamy egg-free Zabaglione

200g/1 cup soy yoghurt
½ cup coconut cream
½ cup coconut oil
Marsala (Optional)
Marsala is a fortified wine, so it is low carb.
You can use a tablespoon or two of Marsala,
Blend all of the above ingredients on low so as not to curdle the yoghurt

Tofu berry smoothie

200g/1 cup silken tofu
200g/1 cup frozen berries
100g/1/2 cup coconut cream
Blend all of the above in a blender until smooth

Vegan Jumpstart Keto Diet Plan

Eat this way for up to five days.

Breakfast
Seitan slices fried in olive oil
or
Tofu berry smoothie
Coffee or tea with coconut oil

Snack
handful of soaked nuts or 1oz/30g vegan cheese
2 tb *Creamy chocolate coconut peanut butter*

Lunch
4oz/100g tofu/seitan/vegan bean burger
2 cup/50g veg/salad
2tb/30g coconut oil or olive oil for cooking or dressing

sea salt to taste

Snack
handful of soaked nuts or 1oz/30g vegan cheese
2 tb *Creamy chocolate coconut peanut butter*

Dinner
4oz/100g tofu/seitan/vegan bean burger
2 cup/50g veg/salad
2tb/30g butter/coconut oil for cooking or dressing
sea salt to taste

ReGeneration-X Mobility

We all need some to move. The body is a beautiful machine, built to move. Our Hunter gatherer ancestors didn't sit at a desk all day, or lie around in front of the television supported by a couch. The ReGeneration-X lifestyle does not mean you have to put in hours of your time running or surviving a punishing fitness routine at all hours of the night and day. Use 'em or Lose' em means that if you move enough to take all your joints and muscles through their full range of motion, you will retain and gain function. Mobility is life, and moderate exercise keeps blood flowing to your all your tissue, bones, muscle, nerves and organs bringing oxygen and nutrients. The lymph system needs the pumping action of movement to filter out toxins and waste.

Do you think you have to exercise to get back in shape? Just the idea of "getting back into shape" might keep you sitting on the couch. What if I told you that simple things you do every day, done with slightly more concentration and repetition, would get you into the shape you want?

Going up and down the stairs
Is that staircase getting longer? It is, because your heart is pumping harder to get blood to your muscles. Following the ReGeneration-X

diet and the ReGeneration-X joint mobilization and strengthening routine will have your heart and veins pumping like they did before, turning back time, taking years off your odometer.

Let's talk about those stairs. You may take the escalator in the mall, or the elevator to get up to your office or apartment, thinking, the stairs, that was something I did before I got old and tired. But with one staircase, or one set of 10 steps, you are using several sets of muscles in taking those stairs. You use the same muscles going up and down. Try with one flight, and then when you feel that one flight of stairs is easy, take another, or simply step up those stairs faster. If you feel your heart pounding, slow down, and take the stairs more slowly.

No stairs? How about sitting down, and getting back up again? You can do it a few times, and then take a rest.. sitting down. This movement uses the same muscles used in going up the stairs, only you are working both legs at a time.

Now let's move onto the upper body. Toned arms and shoulders not only look good, but toned muscles protect your joints, and as I mentioned before, improve circulation, enriching your bones and cartilage.

Did you know that carrying the groceries or lugging your laundry was exercise? We've turned the simple act of walking up stairs and getting up from a chair into a workout. Let's do the same with something we all have to do, be it bags of groceries, laundry, a briefcase or a backpack. Your upper body muscles work whenever you are carrying, lifting, vacuuming, sweeping, and even driving

Walk, don't run, in the beginning. It is not the length of time spent exercising that improves mobility and fitness, but the intensity of the movement. A gradual improvement is always better than doing too much. As the weight melts away and you feel more energetic, you will realize that many of the ways you move in going about your day is actually all the kind of movement you need.

A short session joint mobilization routines will increase muscle release, and get the blood flowing to your bones and sinews. It is a great way to start the day, or a great way to take a break from your routine.

The joint mobilization routine takes about 5 minutes.
Start with one hand on a table to support you so you can go through full range of motion for each joint.

These include knee lifts, hip, knee, ankle and shoulder rotations, spine extensions and rotations. All you need for large joint mobilization.

1.Lift your knee as high as your waist ten times.
Repeat with the other knee. This gets your blood flowing and takes your hip and knee through its flexing and extension motion.

2. To rotate your hip individually stand with your legs shoulder width apart, bend one leg, and with only the big toe touching, make a large circular motion with the thigh, circling in both directions.
Repeat with the other leg.

3. Remove your hand from the table to rotate both hips. Stand with your feet shoulder width apart, hands on the waist, rotate your hips ten times in both directions.

4. To rotate your knees, place your feet together, this time putting your hands on your knees. Make a smaller a circular motion with your knees touching, in both directions.

5. Now put your one hand back on the table and place one foot in front of the other, lift heel and rotate ankle ten times in each direction.
Repeat with other foot.

6 To rotate shoulders stand with your feet shoulder width apart, hands on your waist or arms halfway extended, knees slightly bent, make ten circles forwards and ten backwards.

7. To open release the joints in the spine place your feet together,

knees slightly bent, bend forward head first, following with your torso, and let your arms hang forward. Bend down as much as you can without forcing. Then bend and straighten your knees ten times.

8. To rotate your spine, stand straight, feet together, with your hands gently touching your thighs. Turn first your hips, then torso, then head to look behind, slowly breathing out, breath in and return to the center. Now turn to the other side, alternating ten times.

The strengthening routine takes about 5 minutes. Do these exercises with one hand on a table.

Lower body
1. Knee raises.
Pull your knee to your chest, or as high as possible, ten times each leg, contracting your stomach muscles as you lift your knee.
2 Leg raises. Extend your straightened leg forward as far as you can ten times. Then do the same with the other leg.

3 Backward leg raises. Extend your straightened leg backwards, ten times, then repeat with your other leg.

4. Side ways leg raises. Extend your straightened leg out sideways ten times, then repeat with the other leg.

5. Inward leg raises, pull leg to other side of your body as far as you can then come back to center ten times. Repeat with other leg.

6. Table squats. Holding onto the table, bend your knees as far as you can and come up, ten times.

Upper body
1. Table pushups. Place your hands shoulder width apart, with your arms extended. Keeping your back straight, lower your chest towards the table by bending your elbows ten times.

2. Standing feet shoulder width apart, arms extended out to the side, elbows shoulder height, bend forearms in from elbows inhaling, then extend forearms out to sides to straighten arms, opening chest slowly

breathing out ten times.

3. With your feet shoulder width apart, bend over keeping your back straight. Then extend both arms behind you. Keeping your elbows raised as high as you can, bend your forearms, breathing in, and then extend them behind you breathing out. Repeat this ten times.

Pierre Mattia

My personal experience of a Health Revolution using the ReGeneration-X diet.

As an ex-cycling champion I have many enduring memories of being at the peak of human fitness, much of mine being of my achievements as a racer who was much older than the rest of the pack.

This memory is one of the many that spurred me on to reclaim my health.

The race

I loved racing on my bike. Pushing my body, and my mind, to the extreme felt like going to places I had never been before; during a race my body would reach a point where it was ready to give in to the pain, with no energy left, empty, but my will and experience taught me how to recuperate, reach a threshold of pain, then continue to the next, and the next and find the strength not only to continue, but even win! What a feeling of accomplishment, and amazement realizing what my body could achieve.

It was not all easy and full of zip. I recall my first big crash when I made 'street pizza' of my legs and hands, the impact on bones that felt like they were being crushed in a grinder. The ache for days and weeks after and unknown bruises and contact blows appearing for days and weeks after as they slowly worked their way out of my body. Crashing is part of racing, and I learned to crash in a way to avoid major injuries, like broken wrists, broken collar bone, etc. In my younger days I trained to fall from the bike on grassy fields, learning how to bend my arm and tuck my head in.

I shaved my legs to recover faster and less painfully from road rashes. That's the term I used for when my thigh was stripped of the skin after falling on asphalt. When falling, my main concern was: can I go on, is my bike o.k.? That was the concern of my buddies as well. That was the power of adrenaline! The ultimate pain killer. That's what I miss most, as well as the camaraderie. Your teammates were there to help you get back in the race after a fall, and in turn I waited for them when they fell, and pushed and pulled to rejoin the group. We all shared the same pain, on the bike we were all alike, and there was a great sense of respect among us. It was humbling to know that even when I was at my best, there was always somebody who could beat me.

One race I remember well was in Central Park, in New York City, on a freezing, wet fall morning. Riding in the rain or snow did not bother me. I liked the added challenge. I found that my sense of awareness and reliance on my skills were heightened when riding in bad weather. The start of the morning was the hardest: I had set up the bike the day before, after the training ride. My Gios Torino looked almost like the day I picked it up from Giorgio Barale in Bordighera, Italy that summer: the Campagnolo components were shining, so were my rims, I was ready! After looking out the window at the wet asphalt I let out some air out of the tubulars and quietly left the apartment on West 93rd Street. Outside was still dark at six in the morning. I rode, spinning lightly to the registration table, running into other riders along the way. After the formalities I rode most of the six mile race loop looking for the danger spots like wet fallen leaves, dangerous because very slippery when wet, broken glass, gravel, pot-holes, etc. Finally the race started punctually at seven, and I immediately felt the tension and stress leaving my body, accompanied by burning lungs and throat, for the effort to stay up front.

The start of a circuit race is always hectic and hard. It's like a sprint because everyone wants to be in the front group, but after that the pace slows down a little, just enough to recuperate energy and start thinking about tactics. That's when two riders decided to attack and jumped away from the field. I felt good, the light rain felt cooling on my burning legs and all my senses were heightened, focused on the breakaway and the riders around me. With two laps to go I decided it was time to bridge to the two riders in front: I pushed harder on the pedals going downhill around the Lasker Rink and Pool and seeing that nobody was following me I gave it all and by the the time I got to West Drive I had joined the breakaway. They were surprised to see me, and not pleased because they tried everything to drop me.

They were buddies and much younger than me. They always trained together, but I had more experience and knew my racing body well. I let them do the work of pulling, always staying close to the wheel in front of me. When we arrived at the bottom of the short climb to the finish line I felt great. They started to sprint at the bottom of the hill, hoping I would give up and be happy with third place, but I patiently followed and passed them both almost on the finish line. I heard people cheering and some of the old timers came to pat me on the back! I gave them hope I guess, because a lot of them felt that having arrived at a certain age did not mean they had to hang their racing gear on the wall.

Years later I remembered how it felt to be in that race: about a month before my hip operation I was sitting down watching TV with my hip doing its end of day ache and bone grind, a nasty combination I must say. The TV switched to the results of a regional bicycle race and I recall saying to myself 'I can do that' then I remembered that I couldn't. It was a down moment and all I saw was the arm chair jock in me with past glories but no future. That I think is when the old irritable voice inside me screamed   'I will be damned if I will let this beat me down, I am one of those guys on the TV!' My mind went back to my first coach and his litany diet, diet, DIET! Diet is training, training is diet, it was time to kick ass (mine) and go head to head with my hip and the up-coming operation.
So it was time to investigate what I could do right now...diet time, but what and how?

In the days when I was cycling, high-protein diets were the choice of professional racers. Over the years I saw various dietary fads come and go, but the old guys who kept going seemed to stick to the high-protein high-fat process. I knew that these diets needed monitoring and that I should seek professional help. I chose professional because after reading half a dozen diets, 30 blogs and what seemed like hours and hours Internet of garbage I realized I needed help with this.

It was the memory of past accomplishments and feelings of joy that led me to this wonderful life change. I recalled my bike racing days as I limped down the road with my cane, some young man on a bike whizzed by me shouting 'out of the way grandpa!'. My first thought was that if I had been on my bike I would have chased after him and showed him how it was done, but then I remembered my hip and the need for an operation and that many of my friends were in similar situations or worse. I was determined to change this, the sympathetic looks from doctors and surgeons with the … 'at your age' comments were insults to me and who I know my self to be. If they could not fix it … well I damn well would! It was time to dig in and fight, just like a bunch sprint at the end of a 100 mile race. I was angry and on a mission. I went looking for answers and solutions and this book is the result of my quest. ReGeneration-X, we of Generation-X are turning the tables on life and hitting back!

New York

I have always had the capability to reinvent myself and changing my eating habits has never been difficult, especially when the benefits were felt immediately. I think I knew from very early on that who we are and what we are is not set in stone, I once heard a friend quote Coco Chanel's comment of 'Life is not about finding yourself. Life is about creating yourself', my experience is that all athletes young and old are people who can create and recreate life given the opportunity.

When I was in New York City I felt like going back to racing bicycles, I was 15 years older than the average member of the cycling club I joined, fatter and in poor shape, but I decided I would change. It's the old athlete's mindset, you still have the ability if the right race is in front of you. So change I did: trained hard, shaved my beard of many years (and my legs), started to pay more attention to my diet, quit smoking and transformed my body into the body of an athlete, with a heart beat of 52 at rest and weighing 155 lbs, and riding an average of 400 miles a week. I was at my peak while being at the point when the others were considering stopping!

At first Central Park was my training ground, and I will never forget that 6.1mile loop that I raced on for many years as a member of the Century Road Club Association. I made unforgettable friends and met incredible athletes who went on to become olympic champions and professional international stars. Training and racing with them was exciting and painful at the same time. I always raced against much younger people, and I loved the fact that I had to work so much more to win.

Years went by. I married, had children, and training and racing became harder and harder. Finally I quit. My body changed and went back to its old, pre-racing shape, so did my diet and my mood.

The operation

The hip was a long term victim of one of the many blows and falls from my racing days. It's the problem with many old athletes, football players, cheer leaders, rowers and martial arts practitioners face. We were competitive in our youth and thought ourselves immortal, yet here I was.

I was determined to get back to a life without pain, especially since my racing days were over at 48, I had started practicing Chau Ka Kung Fu and Taiji and now 68 years old, I was an instructor in both. The pain in my leg, at times unbearable after Kung Fu training, stopped me from working out the way I wanted and teaching had become nearly impossible: I had to have the operation, although I was not too excited about the prospect of spending three to four weeks in a hospital, and then walk on crutches for two months, as every doctor warned me.

I approached this new ordeal like a challenge, a race, and my goal was to win, just like the many races I had won. So I looked to my past to create a new future, what exactly was it I did, what did I remember of how I ate and how I approached life when I raced? To a great extent I allowed the things I knew that worked to guide in the past to guide me in the present.

I also remembered how good it felt to be in great athletic shape, how it bolstered my self-confidence, how I was able to transmit my energy to people around me. I wanted that feeling back! The only way to get it back was through exercise, healthy diet and a healthy body.

On Thursday morning, October 16, I was first on the operating list and eager to get it over with. After the wake up call I had the pleasure of experiencing the insertion of a catheter, after which I was taken to the surgery room, prepped and given an epidural anesthetic along with a second sedative so that I would not feel the sawing and hammering (as I was told by the nurse).

The surgery was absolutely painless and I woke up in the recovery room, where I stayed until Friday morning. Back in my room I was immobilized because of an IV in my left arm and two drainage tubes on my right side.

I was advised by doctor Elizabeth Bright to start taking an amino acid formula and Lugol's solution two days after surgery and I could not wait: I had not taken them for about a week and I could feel the difference: I felt sluggish, tired, not able to sleep well. I started taking them on Friday evening and immediately felt more energetic and alert, my mind clearer and I slept soundly that night. At the same time I refused to take the numerous medications prescribed and distributed every day: Celebrex 200MG at 8am and 8pm daily, Ezomepraz EG 20MG daily at 8am, Paracetamolo MG500 Codein 3 daily, Clexane 4000UI one a day at 8pm.

On Saturday, after the drainage tubes and the IV were taken out, I was helped on crutches, and felt comfortable after a few steps, to the amazement of the physical therapist. I was walking up and down the long hallway and doing Taiji exercises on the huge terrace with a beautiful view of the Mediterranean sea. In other words I was training! Every step up or down the stairs had become exercise, walking on crutches had become another form of training, as I shifted my weight form one to the other. Nurses and doctors were commenting on my very fast recovery with admiration, which made me feel great! They appreciated the fact that I was autonomous from the very beginning, not having to call them every minute to get down from bed or get on it, to to be helped to get dressed, etc.

Seeing these positive results the doctor in charge scheduled my transfer to a physiotherapy clinic nearby ahead of schedule, so the following morning, Monday, I left Pietra Ligure to go to the San Michele Clinic in Albenga. I truly feel that my quick recovery was due to not only to my healthy lifestyle, but also to an amino acid formula, which by now I was taking three times a day, and the four drops a day of Lugol's solution.

My roommate

At the San Michele Clinic I rejoined my roommate from the Santa Corona Hospital, Marco Capone, a very funny man in his early seventies, who had had health problems in the past and whose recovery from my same operation was much slower and painful. Being Italian, his diet was mainly pasta, rice, potatoes, some meat, little fish, and very few greens. The nurses made fun of his stock of food and drinks on the table next to his bed: Cheerios, Sprite, olive oil, red wine, vinegar, cookies of different sorts, crackers, bread, peach tea, dried and fresh fruit, candies, and finally water. By comparison my bedside table looked bare, with the amino acids, the Lugol's solution and a bottle of plain water. I felt sorry for him because, although full of life and wit, his body was suffering from the ills of too much sugar, bad habits and the lack of a will to change. I could see that he was curious about my lifestyle, my way of eating, my Taiji exercises in the morning, and he was wondering out loud why I was moving without the pain that was forcing him to lay in bed and not sleep at night. He even asked me to teach him some Taiji movements and breathing exercises, but, like most older people, gave up immediately saying it was too difficult and he would never learn.

Marco had an incredible sense of humor, and no fear of saying what came to his mind, sometimes to my embarrassment. He had a 'voice' for the nurses when he needed their attention and care that resembled the voice of a five year old child begging for a gelato at dinner time. As soon as the nurses had left he would turn to me saying in a grave, serious tone "ah, I feel so much better now, I think I'll eat a cookie, do you want one?" I would just start laughing and he would join me.

When he had visitors, usually his wife and friends, I tried to stay out of the way, maybe go out for a walk, or just lay in bed, but inevitably they would always ask why I was recovering so much faster than Marco. I wanted to tell them that it was because I was not eating all the junk, the pasta, the bread, the sweets, and I was supplementing with amino acids and iodine, and I had years of Kung Fu and Taiji behind me, but as I am not a doctor nor a preacher, I just credited it to my younger age.

Physiotherapy

We had physiotherapy twice a day, mornings at any time between 9 and 12, afternoons between 3 and 6. The first sessions were mainly to get us used to walking and going up and down stairs with crutches. This is where my years of racing bicycles, Taiji and Chau Ka Kung Fu training became so important: no pain was too big, on the bike I had learnt to suffer quietly, without showing my emotions to other riders, because the moment they saw you in pain they would attack. I felt immediately at ease using crutches, with excellent sense of balance, good breathing, keeping a straight position and looking ahead rather than down to my feet, as Chau Ka Kung Fu had taught me to be rooted and Taiji how to breath properly, remain calm and take control of my body. At the clinic the patients were divided in three groups, with a different code for each: the newly arrived were code 1, and that meant that you were confined to your floor and took all your meals in the room, usually for about 3 or 4 days; code 2 meant that you had to go up to the fourth floor restaurant for all your meals and down to the ground floor for physiotherapy, and finally code 3 allowed you to move freely and use the beautiful outdoor garden for walks and therapy.

On my first day, after my first session with a physiotherapist, I was given a code 3: my years of Chau Ka Kung Fu and Taiji helped my balance, mobility and agility. The exercises lying on my back went very well too, again using my deep breathing Taiji techniques, amazed the physiotherapists so much that every session became a lesson in Taiji and Qi Gong.

By the second day I had added my own routine to the exercises and I was doing Taiji exercises in the garden, using my upper body more than the legs, every morning before physiotherapy, and could not help noticing doctors, nurses and physiotherapists watching me and pointing at me while smoking cigarettes on the lawn, yes I forgot to mention that in Italy most doctors and nurses are heavy smokers! I was also walking up and down the four flights to the restaurant and to the physiotherapy room, avoiding the elevator as much as possible. To walk up and down stairs does not seem much, but do it a few days after a hip replacement operation, and you will understand what a challenge that is. The operation itself is very invasive, even when done routinely: it involves cutting through skin, fascia, muscle and bone, after which you are left with a titanium shaft in your thigh bone, a ceramic femoral head and acetabulum, and the prospect of a long rehabilitation period.

In my mind I went back in time to my racing days and the training it required. The rehabilitation, this new challenge, was a new reason to train, to get in shape again: in order to race well I had to train hard every day, in all weather conditions, pushing my body through the levels of pain. Every movement became an exercise: getting down from bed was the first exercise of the day which at first required thinking, but now it has become my way of getting up: first I sit up straight on the bed, then I turn swiftly holding the weight of my body on my fists, finally I get down putting the weight on both legs 50/50. The hard part for most was to turn raising the body by the strength of the arms, but if done quickly it's not hard, but it is still exercise. Walking with crutches, two at first, then one, was training that involved timing, coordination and some strength in the arms, in order to carefully place 50% of my bodyweight on my good leg and 50% on the crutch when using my injured leg, moving along at the same time. Exercise n° 3 was learning how to climb stairs and go down stairs: good leg first, then crutches, then bad leg, going up, crutches with bad leg first, then good leg going down. After two weeks I was using one crutch, and after a month I walked without, aware of every step, especially going up and down stairs, raising my knee high up when I used the bad leg, and landing on my whole foot.

The cat stance of Chau Ka Kung Fu is the ideal position for tying the shoe laces or putting on the sock on your injured leg: I stand straight, legs slightly apart, and put all my weight on my good leg and bend it as low as I can while resting the bad leg on a chair, then putting on socks or tying up shoelaces is a breeze.

Now, almost three months from my operation, I have recuperated at least 75% of my mobility in the operated leg, I take my dog for brisk long walks three times a day. I have resumed teaching Taiji and Chau Ka Kung Fu (no hard kicks yet!). I feel my positions getting lower and lower with time, so is the power in my leg. What I like the most is that now I have no more pain.

I have decided to join a cycling club in nearby Sanremo. I have not been on a bicycle i twenty years, and I feel that the time has come.

Good Food, Bad Food and Hospital Goo!

The hardest part of my hospitalization was the diet to which you are constricted to as a patient, with virtually little or no choice at all: nowadays Italians love pasta, bread and sweets; I say nowadays because it did not use to be like that: the mediterranean diet consisted of vegetables, fish, goat, wild boar, sheep, rabbit, chicken, olives, figs, olive oil, nuts, lots of herbs, chick peas and chick pea flour, chestnuts and chestnut flour. All these ingredients are still present, but they are no longer the staple food, as they have been replaced by all kinds of pastas, rice, pizzas and focaccia, sweets, Nutella, etc. Water or wine have been replaced by beer, Coca-Cola, and all sorts of sweet drinks and fruit juices. The average school kid has cake and very sweet coffee or fruit juice for breakfast, focaccia or a slice of pizza with a soft drink at snack time, lunch is a panino with prosciutto or salami always with a Coke or similar drink, a few candy bars with fruit juice as an afternoon snack, and finally dinner with pasta, always served with bread, a piece of meat with potatoes and sweets or cake for dessert, the whole thing washed down with more Coca Cola and the ever popular EstaThè (a drink sold in supermarkets and bars consisting of tea, water, corn syrup and artificial flavoring and coloring). Grandparents and parents not only have the same eating habits, but they also smoke. Vegetables? none!

Italian parents, wondering why their kids are hyper or unruly at school, bring them to learn Chau Ka Kung Fu, hoping that it will help them but when they don't see any progress they stop the training, not the bad eating habits, the sweets, the computer, the cellphone.

Breakfast, lunch and dinner at the hospital were a nightmare for me. Breakfast consisted of a piece of coffee cake, or two slices of toasted bread that came prepackaged in plastic, with an individual tin cup of jelly, coffee, fake milk or tea. All the patients loved that breakfast, and one hour later most of them complained they were too tired to do the exercises in physiotherapy! Understandable, given the fact that most patients had not done any form of exercise since children, not necessarily living a sedentary life, but eating the wrong food for years.

In fact one evening at dinner I asked for a double serving of spinach, since I had not had the risotto served as first course, and the patient sitting next to me warned me that eating too much spinach was going to upset my stomach! Probably true if I ate ten pounds of spinach at once. This prevailing mentality made people leave the vegetables on the plate, but not all the carbs and sweets.

My roommate Marco agreed with me about the food, but, being Italian, still did not quite understand how I could survive without pasta, bread, cake and croissants. My morning routine was to skip the breakfast of melba toast and jelly, and walk the two flights down to the café where I would meet Marco, my roommate, who took the elevator down, and have a cappuccino with a plain yogurt, which the barmaid had ordered especially for me, as Italians preferred the flavored and sweet kind. It was not much of a breakfast, or at least not as nourishing as the one I was accustomed to at home, but it had to do.

I had lunch and dinner in the mess-hall upstairs, avoiding the usual pastas, risottos, starches in general, and just consuming the little protein served along with the few greens: the result is that I felt undernourished, but knowing that it was just for a few days, I was able to stick to my ketogenic diet for the most part. Some of the nurses and doctors were curious about my habits and questioned me, but had nothing to reproach simply by looking at my daily blood and urine test results.

As I was being dismissed, the head nurse came by to say goodbye and told me that they had never had a patient like me. That was a compliment that made me very happy.

Go on, get fit, eat eggs and bacon!

At seventy years of age I don't want to stop, I have energy to burn, I am never bored, I am a Chau Ka Kung Fu and Taiji instructor, I translate manual and books from English into Italian, and as soon the weather is warmer I am joining one of the local Cycling Clubs.

Most of my childhood friends are dying or are dead; people my age or a couple years older, and all because of cancer. Thanks to my lifestyle and diet I know I am not sick nor about to die. I see old friends still alive resigned to their poor condition and blaming it on old age. It's a lie: they choose not to get healthy and refuse to make the necessary changes. Is it ignorance or just laziness? It just makes me mad as I know that the answer is so simple.

As I don't hunt, like my ancestors did, I still need to sweat and get my heart rate going fast, sweat, ache from exhaustion, this is my hunting, I ride my bike. When I ride for 60 kilometers I am exhausted at the end, knowing that I have given everything. I know now that eating the way I eat helps me and I feel stronger physically and mentally than when I was younger, training and racing bicycles.

I feel I have been able to slow down the aging process through a healthy diet and exercise, believing that I never stop learning and changing.

After being on a ketogenic diet I found that my endurance increased greatly, and the other day, while cycling with a friend, my partner bonked and could not pull any more, he was exhausted although one hour earlier he had told me that he had eaten a big dish of pasta for lunch and felt great! So why did he bonk? On the other hand I felt strong and pulled all the way back home, all along thanking my bacon and eggs for breakfast, fatty fish and salad for lunch, amino acids and coconut oil before cycling. Alas, when I try to explain the benefits of eating fats to my colleagues all I get is a suspicious blank look: after years of false information it is too hard to comprehend. Living in Italy can be very frustrating at times for a person who believes in the benefits of the ketogenic diet: pasta, pizza and sweets rule here! When I tell my grocer that I eat bacon and eggs every day he rolls his eyes and probably he is surprised that I am still alive.

I love double cream! and bacon, and lard, and since I have gone back to eating these fats I have found new levels of energy. When I found out I could eat those foods the ketogenic diet was not so hard for me. My favorite meal of the day is my breakfast of eggs and bacon. My mind is clear and I have gone back to sports, rejecting the idea that old age brings handicapping illnesses. When I read Doctor Roderick Lane's Adam and Eve and started following Doctor Elizabeth Bright's advice, who put me on a ketogenic diet, my life changed. I found my new diet so tasty and satisfying that I had no problem in stopping eating pasta, bread, fruit, sweets, and my stomach never feels "heavy" after a meal. When I see my new self, almost 40 pounds lighter, and still losing, and compare it to before, I am amazed and wonder why other people are not doing it. It's so simple, it just takes determination and common sense. Knowing that I am capable of making these life-changing choices gives me a mental boost and the confidence in myself that I had lost.

This is how I eat most days

Breakfast: two eggs and 3-4 slices of fatty bacon,or lardo pancettato, coffee with butter and coconut oil

Lunch: A big green salad dressed with olive oil, with either a can of mackerel made into a salad with mayo, salt and pepper, or salami or head cheese

Dinner: A fresh green vegetable, with a wild salmon steak, or a grass-fed beefsteak, or fried fresh anchovies, or a bacon cheeseburger. I usually have two glasses of wine with dinner.

I'm never hungry until mealtime. If I train I will take some nuts, pork rinds or some protein powder with me.

I am writing this few pages hoping to inspire those of my age and older, who believe that when they reach a certain age, they stop doing the things that made them happy when they were younger, believing that they are too old or that they will never learn, so they give up and grow old and sick before their time. I don't know many people my age who don't take pills every day to lower their blood pressure or their cholesterol, who constantly have headaches, fevers and colds, etc.

I don't remember the last time I had a cold or the flu and I don't take any medication at all. I follow a ketogenic diet, amino acids daily and a few drops of Lugol's Solution five days a week. My libido is great, I sleep soundly and without interruptions, something I was not able to do for years.
Back on the bike!

Since we moved to Sanremo I rediscovered cycling as a form of exercise. I am taking advantage of the 20-mile bicycle road right behind our building. I cleaned and oiled an old bike I had, very heavy at more than 20 kilos and I have been hitting the road. The one-speed heavy bike makes me work harder and when it hurts I think of when I used to race and the pain becomes minimal. I use my experience and never stop pedaling, always spinning at the same cadence and pushing at the end of the ride, sometimes trying to keep up with the riders who pass me by. I found the fun in riding again and I understand why I loved it in the first place.

Just came back from a bike ride, and in the words of the famous Italian champion Giuseppe Saronni "I feel the power coming back to my legs".

Welcome to the last section

Having read this book and planned some rather wonderful meals and lovelier deserts you have walked with the caveman, from the past into a healthy long future. You have looked to the past to construct the future you deserve. This book and the ReGeneration-X.com website is a universal resource for you and your family, pick it up, put it down and read it a hundred times. Each time you will understand more in your quest for life, happiness and health. Happy ketogenic eating.

Don't degenerate, age backward - REGENERATE!

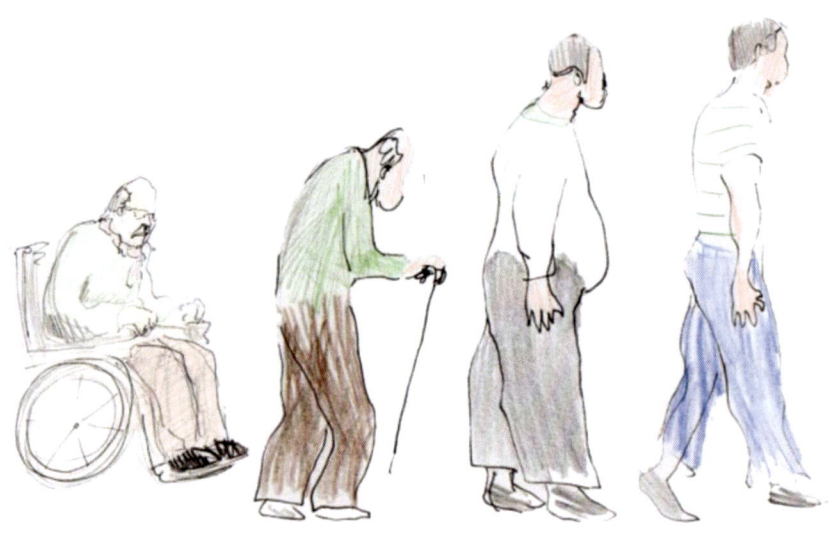

Roderick and Elizabeth the Naturopaths.
The scientific bit

To make this easier for the scientifically inclined, we have adopted the more unusual position of posting webpages that show the efficacy of ketogenics in the conditions listed below. The amount of scientific evidence available online is growing daily, if you include the statements by those who benefit from a ketogenic diet there is a tidal wave of evidence that supports its use. Sadly many of the medical community are still against dietary and health control being given back to the clients; they adhere to the position that everything should be controlled by medication.

This book can be used along similar lines though it is targeted at Generation-X adults wishing to reclaim their vitality.

You will see when you read the reports on ketogenic diet use that there is considerable crossover on all of the conditions mentioned below. It may well be that this simple, tasty and filling diet will be the only shift you will need to reclaim your health across a broad spectrum of supposedly 'age-related conditions'.

Below is a list of drugs that are routinely prescribed in the UK and western world. The list has an accompanying explanation of what they do. You will find that many of these drugs can replaced by the ReGeneration-X diet under the supervision of a Naturopath or physician who has been appropriately trained in the process of using ketogenics. Please check ReGeneration-X.com website for your nearest ketogenic trained physician.

Simvastatin
Simvastatin is used along with a proper diet to help lower cholesterol and fats (such as LDL, triglycerides) and raise "good" cholesterol (HDL) in the blood. It belongs to a group of drugs known as "statins." It works by reducing the amount of cholesterol made by the liver.Since this statement entered the public domain it has now been demonstrated that they are very inefficient almost bordering on the useless, yet poor ratios of LDL A and B cholesterols still remain an issue.

Aspirin
Aspirin "thins" the blood and helps prevent blood clots from forming. So it helps prevent heart attack and stroke. There is a risk of stomach problems, including stomach bleeding, for people who take aspirin regularly.

Levothyroxine sodium
Levothyroxine is used to treat an underactive thyroid (hypothyroidism). It replaces or provides more thyroid hormone, which is normally produced by the thyroid gland. Low thyroid hormone levels can occur naturally or when the thyroid gland is injured by radiation/medications or removed by surgery.

The jury is out concerning the thyroid aspect of ketogenics and thyroid. The main reason is that no formal clinical trials have been set up that could be submitted to medical journals. What can be said is that those physicians who use ketogenics in their medical practice find it a very useful tool. It takes 3 enzymes to convert a ketone to energy in the human cell, it takes 27 to convert sugars to useable energy. Ketones are (do the calculation) 766% efficient which means a lessening of same amount of energy expenditure. This alone will improve thyroid function.

Ramipril
Ramipril (Altace) is an ACE inhibitor. ACE stands for angiotensin converting enzyme. Ramipril is used to treat high blood pressure (hypertension) or congestive heart failure, and to improve survival after a heart attack.
You will have seen by now the other citations often mention lower blood pressure as a result of ketogenic diets.

Bendroflumethiazide
Bendroflumethiazide tablets belong to a group of medicines called thiazide diuretics (water tablets). They may be used to reduce fluid retention (edema) particularly in the heart, kidneys, liver or that caused by medication, by increasing the flow of urine. Reduce high blood pressure alone or with other medication.

Pain Killers
Paracetamol (acetaminophen) is a pain reliever and a fever reducer. The exact mechanism of action is not known. Paracetamol is used to treat many conditions such as headache, muscle aches, arthritis, backache, toothaches, colds, and fevers.
Co-codamol consists of a mixture of paracetamol plus codeine

phosphate (a member of the class of drugs called opioid analgesics). In general, co-codamol is used as required to relieve mild-to-moderate pain and to reduce fever, and so is used for the relief of headaches, migraine, toothache, back pain and period pains.

Omeprazole
Omeprazole (Prilosec, Zegerid) belongs to group of drugs called proton pump inhibitors. It decreases the amount of acid produced in the stomach. Omeprazole is used to treat symptoms of gastroesophageal reflux disease (GERD) and other conditions caused by excess stomach acid.

Lansoprazole
Lansoprazole is used to treat and prevent stomach and intestinal ulcers, erosive esophagitis (damage to the esophagus from stomach acid), and other conditions involving excessive stomach acid such as Zollinger-Ellison syndrome (a condition in which a gastrin-secreting tumor or hyperplasia of the islet cells in the pancreas causes overproduction of gastric acid, resulting in recurrent peptic ulcers). The cutting edge of research is now showing that GERD is an inflammatory disorder, not just 'acid excess'.
http://www.newswise.com/articles/view/558821?print-article

Others of interest.
Blood sugar regulation medications
In the 2014-2015 National Diabetes Audit there were 1,894,887 people with diabetes in England and Wales (1,763,446 in 2013-2014). As you can see this is a rising tide.
Glucovance is an oral medication commonly used to treat type 2 diabetes.
Glucovance contains a combination of glyburide and metformin. Glyburide and metformin are both oral diabetes medicines that help control blood sugar levels.
http://www.ncbi.nlm.nih.gov/pmc/articles/PMC1325029/

I have taken this from the above study......

'The LCKD (Low Carbohydrate Ketogenic Diet) improved glycemic control in patients with type 2 diabetes and diabetes medications were discontinued or reduced in most participants. Because the LCKD can be very effective at lowering blood glucose, patients on diabetes medication who use this diet should be under close medical supervision or capable of adjusting their medication'.

Depression
From Wikipedia, the free encyclopedia
Depression is a state of low mood and aversion to activity that can affect a person's thoughts, behavior, feelings and sense of well-being. People with a depressed mood can feel sad, anxious, empty, hopeless, helpless, worthless, guilty, irritable, ashamed or restless. They may lose interest in activities that were once pleasurable, experience loss of appetite or overeating, have problems concentrating, remembering details or making decisions, and may contemplate, attempt or commit suicide. Insomnia, excessive sleeping, fatigue, aches, pains, digestive problems or reduced energy may also be present. Depressed mood is a feature of some psychiatric syndromes such as major depressive disorder, but it may also be a normal reaction to life events such as grief, a symptom of some bodily ailments or a side effect of some drugs and medical treatments.

Notes

1.   http://www.gponline.com/top-10-prescribed-generic-drugs/article/1029048

2. Long-term effects of a ketogenic diet in obese patients.
Dashti HM[1], Mathew TC, Hussein T, Asfar SK, Behbahani A, Khoursheed MA, Al-Sayer HM, Bo-Abbas YY, Al-Zaid NS.
http://www.ncbi.nlm.nih.gov/pubmed/19641727

3. Glucose Metabolism:
Glucose is metabolized, via the E-M or glycolysis pathway in the cytosol. This pathway is shown below and occurs via a number of steps. I have tried to break this down into logical sequence; there are illustrations below of the biochemical pathways.
1. Glucose is converted to glucose-6-phosphate, then to fructose-6-phosphate
2. In the next stage it is converted into fructose-1:6-di-phosphate. (The numbers refer to which carbon atom the phosphate group is attached to).

3. The fructose-1:6-diphosphate then splits into dihydroxy acetone phosphate and glyceraldehyde-3-phosphate, each of which have three carbon atoms.
4. As a result of stage 3, two molecules of glyceraldehyde-3-phosphate are formed and these lead to the production of pyruvic acid which either enters the mitochondria or is converted into lactic acid.

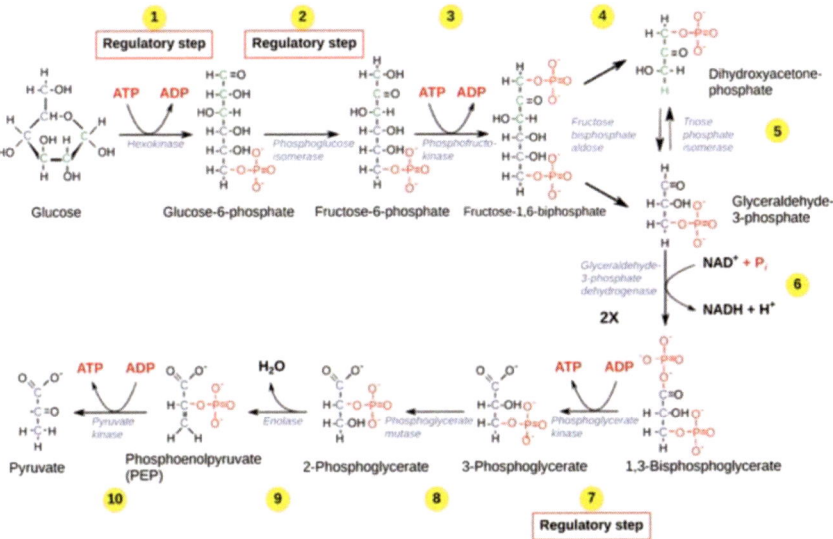

4. Fructose Metabolism:

Fructose has two distinct pathways of metabolism, one in hepatic cells and one in muscle cells. The pathways use different enzymes, but from the perspective of pressure and impact on entry of the metabolites into the mitochondria, the results are similar.

The larger proportion of the fructose ingested is metabolized in the liver where it is converted to fructose-1-phosphate. This is not in the E-M or glycolytic pathway. But it is then converted to glyceraldehyde-3-phosphate and dihydroxy acetone phosphate, just as is glucose. The remaining quantities of the fructose are metabolized by muscle cells. They are converted directly into fructose-6-phosphate, one of the compounds that is in the E-M or glycolysis pathway, just as is glucose. Again, this leads to glyceraldehye-3-phosphate and dihydroxy acetone phosphate, just as is glucose, then on to pyruvic acid. This puts a similar pressure to that of glucose on entry into the mitochondria.

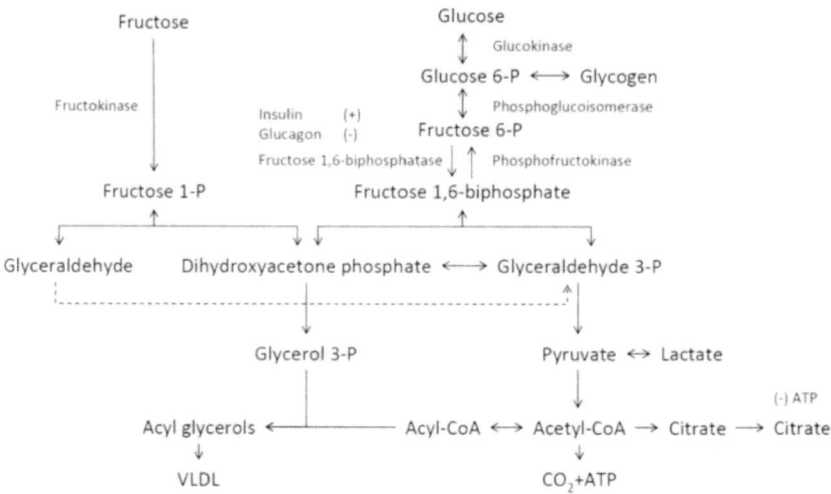

5. 'Long-term fructose intake reduces oxidative defense and alters mitochondrial performance in mice' reported in Nutrition Research,2007; 27(7):423-431
http://www.nrjournal.com/article/S0271-5317(07)00107-8/abstract

6.[Port AM, Ruth MR, Istfan NW. Fructose consumption and cancer: is there a connection? Curr Opin Endocrin Diabetes Obes. 2012;19(5):367-74

7. Haibo Liu, Danshan Huang, David L. McArthur, Laszlo G. Boros, Nicholas Nissen, Anthony P. Heaney. Fructose Induces Transketolase Flux to Promote Pancreatic Cancer Growth. Cancer Res,2010;70(15); 6368–76

8. https://en.wikipedia.org/wiki/Menopause:Wikipedia defines menopause as Menopause, also known as the climacteric, is the time in most women's lives when menstrual periods stop permanently, and the woman is no longer able to have children.[1][2] Menopause typically occurs between 45 and 55 years of age.[1] Medical professionals often define menopause as having occurred when a woman has not had any vaginal bleeding for a year.[3] It may also be defined by a decrease in hormone production by the ovaries.[4] In those who have had surgery to remove the uterus but still have ovaries, menopause may be viewed to have occurred at the time of the surgery or when hormone levels fall.[4] Following the removal of

the uterus, symptoms typically occur earlier, at an average of 45 years of age.[5]

9. https://en.wikipedia.org/wiki/Andropause: Manopause (Andropause) is caused by the reduction of hormones testosterone and dehydroepiandrosterone in middle-aged men. Testosterone assists the male body in building protein and it is crucial for normal sexual drive and stamina. Testosterone also contributes to several metabolic functions including bone formation, and liver function. Andropause is also associated with a decrease in Leydig cells.[3] A steady decline in testosterone levels with age (in both men and women) is well documented.[4]
External factors that can[5] cause testosterone levels to fall include certain forms of medication, poor diet, excessive alcohol consumption, illness, lack of sleep, lack of sex, stress, or surgery. It can also be a symptom of neuroendocrine dysfunction after a mild traumatic brain injury.

References to studies illustrating beneficial effects of the ketogenic diet on illnesses

Cancer:
Klement RJ and Kämmerer U: Is there a role for carbohydrate restriction in the treatment and prevention of cancer? Nutr Metab (Lond) 8: 75, 2011

Vaughn AE and Deshmukh M: Glucose metabolism inhibits apoptosis in neurons and cancer cells by redox inactivation of cytochrome c. Nat Cell Biol 10: 1477-1483, 2008.

Gunter MJ, Hoover DR, Yu H, Wassertheil-Smoller S, Rohan TE, Manson JE, Li J, Ho GY, Xue X, Anderson GL, et al: Insulin, insulin-like growth factor-I, and risk of breast cancer in postmenopausal women. J Natl Cancer Inst 101: 48-60, 2009.

Paoli A, Rubini A, Volek JS and GrimaldiKA: Beyond weight loss: A review of the therapeutic uses of very-low-carbohydrate (ketogenic) diets. Eur J Clin Nutr 67: 789-796, 2013.

Ruskin DN and Masino SA: The nervous system and metabolic dysregulation: Emerging evidence converges on ketogenic diet therapy. Front Neurosci 6: 33, 2012.

Jansen, N., Walach, H.''The development of tumours under a ketogenic diet in association with the novel tumour marker TKTL1: A case series in general practice''. Oncology Letters 11.1 (2016): 584-592.

Schwaab J, Horisberger K, Ströbel P, Bohn B, Gencer D, Kähler G, Kienle P, Post S, Wenz F, Hofmann WK, et al: Expression of Transketolase like gene 1 (TKTL1) predicts disease-free survival in patients with locally advanced rectal cancer receiving neoadjuvant chemoradiotherapy. BMC Cancer 11: 363, 2011.

Zhang S, Yang JH, Guo CK and Cai PC: Gene silencing of TKTL1 by RNAi inhibits cell proliferation in human hepatoma cells. Cancer Lett 253: 108-114, 2007

Diabetes

Klein S, Sheard NF, Pi-Sunyer S, Daly A, Wylie-Rosett J, Kulkarni K, Clark NG. Weight management through lifestyle modification for the prevention and management of type 2 diabetes: rationale and strategies. A statement of the American Diabetes Association, the North American Association for the Study of Obesity, and the American Society for Clinical Nutrition. Am J Clin Nutr. 2004;80:257–263.

Arora SK, McFarlane SI. The case for low carbohydrate diets in diabetes management. Nutr Metab (Lond) 2005;2:16. doi: 10.1186/1743-7075-2-16.

Osler W, McCrae T. The Principles and Practice of Medicine. New York, Appleton and Co.; 1923.

Allen FM, Stillman E, Fitz R. Total dietary regulation in the treatment of diabetes: monograph No. 11. New York, The Rockefeller Institute for Medical Research; 1919.

Stern L, Iqbal N, Seshadri P, Chicano KL, Daily DA, McGrory J, Williams M, Gracely EJ, Samaha FF. The effects of low-carbohydrate versus conventional weight loss diets in severely obese adults: one-year follow-up of a randomized trial. Ann Intern Med. 2004;140:778–785.

Samaha FF, Iqbal N, Seshadri P, Chicano K, Daily D, McGrory J, Williams T, Williams M, Gracely EJ, Stern L. A low-carbohydrate as compared with a low-fat diet in severe obesity. N Engl J Med. 2003;348:2074–2081. doi: 10.1056/NEJMoa022637.

Gannon MC, Nuttall FQ. Effect of a high-protein, low-carbohydrate diet on blood glucose control in people with type 2 diabetes. Diabetes. 2004;53:2375–2382.

Boden G, Sargrad K, Homko C, Mozzoli M, Stein TP. Effect of a low-carbohydrate diet on appetite, blood glucose levels, and insulin resistance in obese patients with type 2 diabetes. Ann Intern Med. 2005;142:403–411.

Nielsen JV, Jonsson E, Nilsson AK. Lasting improvement of hyperglycaemia and bodyweight: low-carbohydrate diet in type 2 diabetes. A brief report. Ups J Med Sci. 2005;110:179–183.

Yancy WS, Jr, Vernon MC, Westman EC. Brief report: a pilot trial of a low-carbohydrate, ketogenic diet in patients with type II diabetes. Metabolic Syndrome and Related Disorders. 2003;1:239–244. doi: 10.1089/154041903322716723.

The Atkins Trial Kit Handbook: A Simple Guide to Doing Atkins. Ronkonkoma, NY, Atkins Nutritionals, Inc.; 2001.

Durnin JVGA, Womersley J. Body fat assessed from total body density and its estimation from skinfold thickness: measurements on 481 men and women aged from 16 to 72 years. Br J Nutr. 1974;32:77–97. doi: 10.1079/BJN19740060.

Sharman MJ, Gomez AL, Kraemer WJ, Volek JS. Very low-carbohydrate and low-fat diets affect fasting lipids and postprandial lipemia differently in overweight men. J Nutr. 2004;134:880–885.

Volek JS, Sharman MJ, Gomez AL, DiPasquale C, Roti M, Pumerantz A, Kraemer WJ. Comparison of a very low-carbohydrate and low-fat diet on fasting lipids, LDL subclasses, insulin resistance, and postprandial lipemic responses in overweight women. J Am Coll Nutr. 2004;23:177–184.

Meckling KA, O'Sullivan C, Saari D. Comparison of a low-fat diet to a low-carbohydrate diet on weight loss, body composition, and risk factors for diabetes and cardiovascular disease in free-living, overweight men and women. J Clin Endocrinol Metab. 2004;89:2717–2723. doi: 10.1210/jc.2003-031606.

Volek JS, Sharman MJ, Love DM, Avery NG, Gomez AL, Scheett TP, Kraemer WJ. Body composition and hormonal responses to a carbohydrate-restricted diet. Metabolism. 2002;51:864–870. doi: 10.1053/meta.2002.32037.

Denke MA. Metabolic effects of high-protein, low-carbohydrate diets. Am J Cardiol. 2001;88:59–61. doi: 10.1016/S0002-9149(01)01586-7.

Yancy WS, Jr, Olsen MK, Guyton JR, Bakst RP, Westman EC. A low-carbohydrate, ketogenic diet versus a low-fat diet to treat obesity and hyperlipidemia: a randomized, controlled trial. Ann Intern Med. 2004;140:769–777.

Vernon MC, Mavropoulos J, Yancy WS, Jr, Westman EC. Brief report: clinical experience of a carbohydrate-restricted diet: effect on diabetes mellitus. Metabolic Syndrome and Related Disorders. 2003;1:233–238. doi: 10.1089/154041903322716714.

Intensive blood-glucose control with sulphonylureas or insulin compared with conventional treatment and risk of complications in patients with type 2 diabetes (UKPDS 33). UK Prospective Diabetes Study (UKPDS) Group. Lancet. 1998;352:837–853. doi: 10.1016/S0140-6736(98)07019-6.

Purnell JQ, Hokanson JE, Marcovina SM, Steffes MW, Cleary PA, Brunzell JD. Effect of excessive weight gain with intensive therapy of type 1 diabetes on lipid levels and blood pressure: results from the DCCT. Diabetes Control and Complications Trial. JAMA. 1998;280:140–146. doi: 10.1001/jama.280.2.140.

Westman EC, Yancy WS, Edman JS, Tomlin KF, Perkins CE. Effect of six-month adherence to a very-low-carbohydrate diet program. Am J Med. 2002;113:30–36. doi: 10.1016/S0002-9343(02)01129-4.

Yancy WS, Jr, Boan J. Patient Treatment Adherence: Concepts, Interventions, and Measurement. Mahwah, NJ, Lawrence Erlbaum Associates, Inc.; 2005. Adherence to Diet Recommendations.

Obesity

Bray GA. Medical consequences of obesity. J Clin Endocrinol Metab. 2004;89:2583–9.

Grundy SM, Barnett JP. Metabolic and health complications of obesity. Dis Mon. 1990;36:641–731.

Pi-Sunyer FX. Medical hazards of obesity. Ann Intern Med. 1993;119:655–60.

Simopoulos AP, Van Itallie TB. Body weight, health, and longevity. Ann Intern Med. 1984;100:285–95.

McGinnis JM, Foege WH. Actual causes of death in the United States. JAMA. 1993;270:2207–12.

Thomas PR, editor. Washington: National Academy Press; 1995. Weighing the Options: Criteria for Evaluating Weight-Management Programs.

Andersen T, Stokholm KH, Backer OG, Quaade F. Long-term (5-year) results after either horizontal gastroplasty or very-low-calorie diet for morbid obesity. Int J Obes. 1988;12:277–84.

Kramer FM, Jeffery RW, Forster JL, Snell MK. Long-term follow-up of behavioral treatment for obesity: Patterns of regain among men and women. Int J Obes. 1989;13:123–36.

Peni MG. Improving maintenance of weight loss following treatment by diet and lifestyle modification. In: Wadden TA, Van Itallie TB, editors. Treatment of the Seriously Obese Patient. New York: Guilford; 1992. pp. 456–77.

Sondike SB, Copperman N, Jacobson MS. Effects of a low-carbohydrate diet on weight loss and cardiovascular risk factors in overweight adolescents. J Pediatr. 2003;142:253–8.

Yancy WS, Jr, Guyton JR, Bakst RP, Westman EC. A randomized, controlled trial of a low-carbohydrate ketogenic diet versus a low-fat diet for obesity and hyperlipidemia. Am J Clin Nutr. 2002;72:343S.

Dashti HM, Bo-Abbas YY, Asfar SK, et al. Ketogenic diet modifies the risk factors of heart disease in obese patients. Nutrition. 2003;19:901–2.

Wilder RM. The effect of ketonemia on the course of epilepsy. Mayo Clin Proc. 1921;2:307–8.

Pilkington TR, Rosenoer VM, Gainsborough H, Carey M. Diet and weight-reduction in the obese. Lancet. 1960;i:856–8.

Howard BV, Wylie-Rosett J. Sugar and cardiovascular disease: A statement for healthcare professionals from the Committee on Nutrition of the Council on Nutrition, Physical Activity, and Metabolism of the American Heart Association. Circulation. 2002;106:523–7. Erratum in 2003;107:2166.

Franceschi S, Favero A, Decarli A, et al. Intake of macronutrients and risk of breast cancer. Lancet. 1996;347:1351–6.

Liu S, Manson JE, Stantpfer MJ, et al. Dietary glycemic load assessed by food-frequency questionnaire in relation to plasma high-density-lipoprotein cholesterol and fasting plasma triacylglycerols in postmenopausal women. Am J Clin. 2001;73:560–6.

Gaziano JM, Hennekens CH, O'Donnell CJ, Breslow JL, Buring JE. Fasting triglycerides, high-density lipoprotein and risk of myocardial infarction. Circulation. 1997;96:2520–5.

Kreitzman SN. Factors influencing body composition during very-low-caloric diets. Am J Clin Nutr. 1992;56(1 Suppl):217S–23S.

Mitchell GA, Kassovska-Bratinova S, Boukaftane Y, et al. Medical aspects of ketone body metabolism. Clin Invest Med. 1995;18:193–216.

Koeslag JH. Post-exercise ketosis and the hormone response to exercise: A review. Med Sci Sports Exerc. 1982;14:327–34.

Winder WW, Baldwin KM, Holloszy JO. Exercise-induced increase in the capacity of rat skeletal muscle to oxidize ketones. Can J Physiol Pharmacol. 1975;53:86–91.

Yehuda S, Rabinovitz S, Mostofsky DI. Essential fatty acids are mediators of brain
biochemistry and cognitive functions. J Neurosci Res. 1999;56:565–70.

Amiel SA. Organ fuel selection: Brain. Proc Nutr Soc. 1995;54:151–5.

Singhi PD. Newer antiepileptic drugs and non surgical approaches in epilepsy. Indian J Pediatr. 2000;67:S92–8.

Janigro D. Blood-brain barrier, ion homeostatis and epilepsy: Possible implications towards the understanding of ketogenic diet mechanisms. Epilepsy Res. 1999;37:223–32.

Kossoff EH, Pyzik PL, McGrogan JR, Vining EP, Freeman JM. Efficacy of the ketogenic diet for infantile spasms. Pediatrics. 2002;109:780–3.

El-Mallakh RS, Paskitti ME. The ketogenic diet may have mood-stabilizing properties. Med Hypotheses. 2001;57:724–6.

Ziegler DR, Araujo E, Rotta LN, Perry ML, Goncalves CA. A ketogenic diet increases protein phosphorylation in brain slices of rats. J Nutr. 2002;132:483–7.

Cullingford TE, Eagles DA, Sato H. The ketogenic diet upregulates expression of the gene encoding the key ketogenic enzyme mitochondrial 3-hydroxy-3-methylglutaryl-CoA synthase in rat brain. Epilepsy Res. 2002;49:99–107.

Prentice AM. Manipulation of dietary fat and energy density and subsequent effects on substrate flux and food intake. Am J Clin Nutr. 1998;67(3 Suppl):535S–41S.

Foster GD, Wyatt HR, Hill JO, et al. A randomized trial of a low-carbohydrate diet for obesity. N Engl J Med. 2003;348:2082–90.

He K, Merchant A, Rimm EB, et al. Dietary fat intake and risk of stroke in male US healthcare professionals: 14 year prospective cohort study. BMJ. 2003;327:777–82.

Westman EC, Mavropoulos J, Yancy WS, Volek JS. A review of low-carbohydrate ketogenic diets. Curr Atheroscler Rep. 2003;5:476–83.

Petersen KF, Befroy D, Dufour S, et al. Mitochondrial dysfunction in the elderly: Possible role in insulin resistance. Science. 2003;300:1140–2.

Foster-Powell K, Holt SH, Brand-Miller JC. International table of glycemic index and glycemic load values: 2002. Am J Clin Nutr. 2002;76:5–56.

Leeds AR. Glycemic index and heart disease. Am J Clin Nutr. 2002;76:286S–9S.

Liu S, Willett WC, Stampfer MJ, et al. A prospective study of dietary glycaemic load, carbohydrate intake, and risk of coronary heart disease in US women. Am J Clin Nutr. 2000;71:1455–61.

Sims EA, Danford E, Jr, Horton ES, Bray GA, Glennon JA, Salans LB. Endocrine and metabolic effects of experimental obesity in man. Recent Prog Horm Res. 1973;29:457–96.

Golay A, DeFronzo RA, Ferrannini E, et al. Oxidative and non-oxidative glucose metabolism in non-obese type 2 (non-insulin dependent) diabetic patients. Diabetologia. 1988;31:585–91.

Defronzo RA, Simonson D, Ferrannini E. Hepatic and peripheral insulin resistance: A common feature of type 2 (non-insulin-dependent) and type 1 (insulin-dependent) diabetes mellitus. Diabetologia. 1982;23:313–9.

Defronzo RA, Diebert D, Hendler R, Felig P. Insulin sensitivity and insulin binding in maturity onset diabetes. J Clin Invest. 1979;63:939–46.

Hollenbeck B, Y-Di Chen, Reaven GM. A comparison of the relative effects of obesity and non-insulin dependent diabetes mellitus on in vivo insulin-stimulated glucose utilization. Diabetes. 1984;33:622–6.

Kolterman OG, Gray RS, Griffin J, et al. Receptor and postreceptor defects contribute to the insulin resistance in noninsulin-dependent diabetes mellitus. J Clin Invest. 1981;68:957–69.

Gresl TA, Colman RJ, Roecker EB, et al. Dietary restriction and glucose regulation in aging rhesus monkeys: A follow-up report at 8.5 yr. Am J Physiol Endocrinol Metab. 2001;281:E757–65.

Hansen BC, Bodkin NL. Primary prevention of diabetes mellitus by prevention of obesity in monkeys. Diabetes. 1993;42:1809–14.

Coulston AM, Liu GC, Reaven GM. Plasma glucose, insulin and lipid responses to high-carbohydrate low-fat diets in normal humans. Metabolism. 1983;32:52–6.

Chen YDI, Swami S, Skowronski R, Coulston AM, Reaven GM.

Effects of variations in dietary fat and carbohydrate intake on postprandial lipemia in patients with non-insulin dependent diabetes mellitus. J Clin Endocrinol Metab. 1993;76:347–51.

Chen YD, Hollenbeck CB, Reaven GM, Coulston AM, Zhou MY. Why do low-fat high-carbohydrate diets accentuate postprandial lipemia in patients with NIDDM? Diabetes Care. 1995;18:10–6.

Gardner CD, Kraemer HC. Monosaturated versus polyunsaturated dietary fat and serum lipids and lipoproteins. Arterioscler Thromb Vasc Biol. 1995;15:1917–25.

Jeppesen J, Schaaf P, Jones C, Zhoue MY, Chen YD, Reaven GM. Effects of low-fat, high-carbohydrate diets on risk factors for ischemic heart disease in post-menopausal women. Am J Clin Nutr. 1997;65:1027–33.

Mensink RP, Katan MN. Effect of dietary fatty acids on serum lipids and lipoproteins. Arterioscler Thromb. 1992;12:911–9.

Groot PH, Van Stiphout WA, Krauss XH, et al. Postprandial lipoprotein metabolism in normolipidemic men with and without coronary artery disease. Arterioscler Thromb. 1991;11:653–62.

Patsch JR, Miesenbock G, Hopferweiser T, et al. Relation of triglyceride metabolism and coronary artery disease studies in the postprandial state. Arterioscler Thromb. 1992;12:1336–45.

Abbasi F, McLaughlin T, Lamendola C, et al. High carbohydrate diets, triglyceride-rich lipoproteins and coronary heart disease risk. Am J Cardiol. 2000;85:45–8.

Sharman MJ, Kraemer WJ, Love DM, et al. A ketogenic diet favorably affects serum biomarkers for cardiovascular disease in normal-weight men. J Nutr. 2002;132:1879–85.

Mohanty P, Hamouda W, Garg R, Aljada A, Ghanim H, Dandona P. Glucose challenge stimulates reactive oxygen species (ROS) generation by leucocytes. J Clin Endocrinol Metab. 2000;85:2970–3.

Kaaks R. Nutrition and colorectal cancer risk: The role of insulin and insulin-like growth factor-1. European Conference on Nutrition and Cancer. International Agency for Research on Cancer and Europe Against Cancer Programme of the European Commission; Lyon, France. June 21 to 21; 2001. A0.14. (Abst)

Berrino F, Bellati C, Oldani S, et al. DIANA trial on diet and endogenous hormones. European Conference on Nutrition and Cancer. International Agency for Research on Cancer and Europe Against Cancer Programme of the European Commission; Lyon, France. June 21 to 24; 2001. A0.27. (Abst)

Willett WC. Cancer prevention: Diet and risk reduction: Fat. In: DeVita V, Hellman S, Rosenberg S, editors. Cancer: Principles and Practice of Oncology. 5th edn. New York: Lippincott-Raven; 1997. pp. 559–66.

Fearon KC. Nutritional pharmacology in the treatment of neoplastic disease. Baillieres Clin Gastroenterol. 1988;2:941–9.

Wolf RL, Cauley JA, Baker CE, et al. Factors associated with calcium absorption efficiency in pre- and perimenopausal women. Am J Clin Nutr. 2000;72:466–71.

Brehm BJ, Seeley RI, Daniels SR, D'Alessio DA. A randomized trial comparing a very low carbohydrate diet and a calorie-restricted low fat diet on body weight and cardiovascular risk factors in healthy women. J Clin Endocrinol Metab. 2003;88:1617–23.

Samaha FF, Iqbal N, Seshadri P, et al. A low-carbohydrate as compared with a low-fat diet in severe obesity. N Engl J Med. 2003;348:2074–81.

Polycystic Ovary Syndrome

Azziz R, Woods KS, Reyna R, Key TJ, Knochenhauer ES, Yildiz BO: The prevalence and features of the polycystic ovary syndrome in unselected population. J Clin Endocrinol Metab. 2004, 89: 2745-9.

10.1210/jc.2003-032046.

Dunaif A, Graf M, Mandeli J, Laumas V, Dobrjansky A: Characterization of groups of hyperandrogenic women with acanthosis nigricans, impaired glucose tolerance, and/or hyperinsulinemia. J Clin Endocrinol Metab. 1987, 65: 499-507.

Ehrmann DA: Medical progress. Polycystic ovary syndrome. NEJM. 2005, 352: 1223-36. 10.1056/NEJMra041536.

Dunaif A: Insulin resistance and the polycystic ovary syndrome: mechanism and implications for pathogenesis. Endocr Rev. 1997, 18: 774-800. 10.1210/er.18.6.774.

Legro RS, Kunselman AR, Dodson WC, Dunaif A: Prevalence and predictors of risk for type 2 diabetes mellitus and impaired glucose tolerance in polycystic ovary syndrome: a prospective, controlled study in 254 affected women. J Clin Endocrinol Metab. 1999, 84: 165-9. 10.1210/jc.84.1.165.

Burghen G, Givens J, Kitabachi A: Correlation of hyperandrogenism with hyperinsulinism in polycystic ovarian disease. J Clin Endocrinol Metab. 1980, 50: 113-6.

Glueck CJ, Moreira A, Goldenberg N, Sieve L, Wang P: Pioglitazone and metformin in obese women with PCOS not optimally responsive to metformin. Hum Reprod. 2003, 18: 1618-25. 10.1093/humrep/deg343.

Chou KH, von Eye Corleta H, Capp E, Spritzer PM: Clinical, metabolic, and endocrine parameters in response to metformin in obese women with polycystic ovary syndrome: a randomized, double-blind and placebo-controlled trial. Horm Metab Res. 2003, 35: 86-91. 10.1055/s-2003-39056.

Velazquez EM, Mendoza S, Hamer T, Sosa F, Glueck CJ: Metformin therapy in polycystic ovary syndrome reduces hyperinsulinemia, insulin resistance, hyperandrogenemia, and systolic blood pressure, while facilitating normal menses and pregnancy. Metabolism. 1994,

43: 647-54. 10.1016/0026-0495(94)90209-7.

Dunaif A, Scott D, Finegood D, Quintana B, Whitcomb R: The insulin-sensitizing agent troglitazone improves metabolic and reproductive abnormalities in the polycystic ovary syndrome. J Clin Endocrinol Metab. 1996, 81: 3299-306. 10.1210/jc.81.9.3299.

Nestler JE, Jakubowicz DJ, de Vargas AF, Brik C, Quintero N, Medina F: Insulin stimulates testosterone biosynthesis by human thecal cells fromwomen with polycystic ovarian syndrome by activating its own receptor and using inositolglycan mediators as the signal transduction system. J Clin Endocrinol Metab. 1998, 83: 2001-5. 10.1210/jc.83.6.2001.

Nestler JE, Jakubowicz DJ, Reamer P, Gunn RD, Allan G: Ovulatory and metabolic effects of d-chiro-inositol in the polycystic ovary syndrome. NEJM. 1999, 340: 1314-20. 10.1056/NEJM199904293401703.

Barbieri RL, Makris A, Randall RW, Daniels G, Kistner RW, Ryan KJ: Insulin stimulates androgen accumulation in incubations of ovarian stroma obtained from women with hyperandrogenism. J Clin Endocrinol Metab. 1986, 62: 904-10.

Moran LJ, Noakes M, Clifton PM, Tomlinson L, Norman RJ: Dietary composition in restoring reproductive and metabolic physiology in overweight women with polycystic ovary syndrome. J Clin Endocrinol Metab. 2003, 88: 812-819. 10.1210/jc.2002-020815.

Huber-Buchholz MM, Carey DGP, Norman RJ: Restoration of reproductive potential by lifestyle modification in obese polycystic ovary syndrome: role of insulin sensitivity and luteinizing hormone. J Clin Endocrinol Metab. 1999, 84: 1470-1474. 10.1210/jc.84.4.1470.

Yancy WS, Olsen MK, Guyton JR, Bakst RP, Westman EC: A low-carbohydrate ketogenic diet versus a low-fat diet to treat obesity and hyperlipidemia. Ann Intern Med. 2004, 140: 769-777.

Boden G, Sargrad K, Homko C, Mozzoli M, Stein TP: Effect of a low-carbohydrate diet on appetite, blood glucose levels, and insulin resistance in obese patients with type 2 diabetes. Ann Intern Med. 2005, 142: 403-411.

Atkins RC: Dr. Atkins' New Diet Revolution. 1998, New York, Simon & Schuster

Cronin L, Guyatt G, Griffith L, Wong E, Azziz R, Futterweit W, Cook D, Dunaif A: Development of a health-related quality-of-life questionnaire(PCOSQ) for women with polycystic ovary syndrome (PCOS). J Clin Endocrinol Metab. 1998, 83: 1976-1987. 10.1210/jc.83.6.1976.

Guyatt G, Weaver B, Cronin L, Dooley JA, Azziz R: Health-related quality of life in women with polycystic ovary syndrome, a self-administered questionnaire, was validated. J Clin Epidem. 2004, 57: 1279-1287. 10.1016/j.jclinepi.2003.10.018.

Hays JH, Disabatino A, Gorman RT, Vincent S, Stillabower ME: Effect of a high saturated fat and no-starch diet on serum lipid subfractions in patients with documented atherosclerotic cardiovascular disease. Mayo Clin Proc. 2003, 78: 1331-1336.

Nestler JE, Powers LP, Matt DW, Steingold KA, Plymate SR, Rittmaster RS, Clore JN, Blackard WGB: A direct effect of hyperinsulinemia on serum sex-hormone-binding globulin levels in obese women with the polycystic ovary syndrome. J Clin Endocrinol Metab. 1991, 72: 83-89.

Alzheimer's and Parkinson's

Acheson KJ. Carbohydrate and weight control: where do we stand? Curr Opin Clin Nutr Metab Care. 2004;7:485–492.

al-Mudallal AS, LaManna JC, Lust WD, Harik SI. Diet-induced ketosis does not cause cerebral acidosis. Epilepsia. 1996;37:258–261.

Appleton DB, De Vivo DC. An experimental animal model for the effect of ketogenic diet on epilepsy. Proc Aust Assoc Neurol.

1973;10:75–80.

Barberger-Gateau P, Letenneur L, Deschamps V, Peres K, Dartigues JF, Renaud S. Fish, meat, and risk of dementia: cohort study. BMJ. 2002;325:932–933.

Bellido T, Huening M, Raval-Pandya M, Manolagas SC, Christakos S. Calbindin-D28k is expressed in osteoblastic cells and suppresses their apoptosis by inhibiting caspase-3 activity. J Biol Chem. 2000;275:26328–26332.

Benardo LS. Prevention of epilepsy after head trauma: do we need new drugs or a new approach? Epilepsia. 2003;44 Suppl 10:27–33.

Bough KJ, Gudi K, Han FT, Rathod AH, Eagles DA. An anticonvulsant profile of the ketogenic diet in the rat. Epilepsy Res. 2002;50:313–325.

Bough KJ, Wetherington J, Hassel B, Pare JF, Gawryluk JW, Greene JG, et al. Mitochondrial biogenesis in the anticonvulsant mechanism of the ketogenic diet. Ann Neurol. 2006;60

Cahill GF, Jr, Veech RL. Ketoacids? Good medicine? Trans Am Clin Climatol Assoc. 2003;114:149–161.

Caraballo RH, Cersosimo RO, Sakr D, Cresta A, Escobal N, Fejerman N. Ketogenic diet in patients with Dravet syndrome. Epilepsia. 2005;46:1539–1544.

Chamorro A, Hallenbeck J. The harms and benefits of inflammatory and immune responses in vascular disease. Stroke. 2006;37:291–293.

Chen J, Nagayama T, Jin K, Stetler RA, Zhu RL, Graham SH, Simon RP. Induction of caspase-3-like protease may mediate delayed neuronal death in the hippocampus after transient cerebral ischemia. J Neurosci. 1998;18:4914–4928.

Cherian L, Peek K, Robertson CS, Goodman JC, Grossman RG. Calorie sources and recovery from central nervous system ischemia.

Crit Care Med. 1994;22:1841–1850.

Ciraolo ST, Previs SF, Fernandez CA, Agarwal KC, David F, Koshy J, et al. Model of extreme hypoglycemia in dogs made ketotic with (R,S)-1, 3-butanediol acetoacetate esters. Am J Physiol. 1995;269:E67–E75.

Crumrine PK. Lennox-Gastaut syndrome. J Child Neurol. 2002;17 Suppl 1:S70–S75.

Cullingford TE. The ketogenic diet; fatty acids, fatty acid-activated receptors and neurological disorders. Prostaglandins Leukot Essent Fatty Acids. 2004;70:253–264.

Cunnane SC, Musa K, Ryan MA, Whiting S, Fraser DD. Potential role of polyunsaturates in seizure protection achieved with the ketogenic diet. Prostaglandins Leukot Essent Fatty Acids. 2002;67:131–135.

Dardzinski BJ, Smith SL, Towfighi J, Williams GD, Vannucci RC, Smith MB. Increased plasma beta-hydroxybutyrate, preserved cerebral energy metabolism, and amelioration of brain damage during neonatal hypoxia ischemia with dexamethasone pretreatment. Pediatr Res. 2000;48:248–255.

Desrochers S, David F, Garneau M, Jetté M, Brunengraber H. Metabolism of R- and S-1,3-butanediol in perfused livers from meal-fed and starved rats. Biochem J. 1992;285:647–653.

Desrochers S, Dubreuil P, Brunet J, Jetté M, David F, Landau BR, Brunengraber H. Metabolism of (R,S)-1,3-butanediol acetoacetate esters, potential parenteral and enteral nutrients in conscious pigs. Am J Physiol. 1995;268:E660–E667.

de Lau LM, Bornebroek M, Witteman JC, Hofman A, Koudstaal PJ, Breteler MM. Dietary fatty acids and the risk of Parkinson disease: the Rotterdam study. Neurology. 2005;64:2040–2045.

Duan W, Mattson MP. Dietary restriction and 2-deoxyglucose

administration improve behavioral outcome and reduce degeneration of dopaminergic neurons in models of Parkinson's disease. J Neurosci Res. 1999;57:195–206.

Engelhart MJ, Geerlings MI, Ruitenberg A, van Swieten JC, Hofman A, Witteman JC, Breteler MM. Diet and risk of dementia: does fat matter? The Rotterdam Study. Neurology. 2002;59:1915–1921.

Erecinska M, Nelson D, Daikhin Y, Yudkoff M. Regulation of GABA level in rat brain synaptosomes: fluxes through enzymes of the GABA shunt and effects of glutamate, calcium, and ketone bodies. J Neurochem. 1996;67:2325–2334.

Fraser DD, Whiting S, Andrew RD, Macdonald EA, Musa-Veloso K, Cunnane SC. Elevated polyunsaturated fatty acids in blood serum obtained from children on the ketogenic diet. Neurology. 2003;60:1026–1029.

Freeman J, Veggiotti P, Lanzi G, Tagliabue A, Perucca E. The ketogenic diet: from molecular mechanisms to clinical effects. Epilepsy Res. 2006;68:145–180.

Freeman JM, Vining EP, Pillas DJ, Pyzik PL, Casey JC, Kelly LM. The efficacy of the ketogenic diet – 1998: a prospective evaluation of intervention in 150 children. Pediatrics. 1998;102:1358–1363.

Fujikawa DG. Prolonged seizures and cellular injury: understanding the connection. Epilepsy Behav. 2005;7 Suppl 3:S3–S11.

Garcia O, Massieu L. Strategies for neuroprotection against l-trans-2, 4-pyrrolidine dicarboxylate-induced neuronal damage during energy impairment *in vitro*. J Neurosci Res. 2001;64:418–428.

George AJ, Holsinger RMD, McLean CA, Laughton KM, Beyreuther K, Evin G, et al. APP intracellular domain is increased and soluble A β is reduced with diet-induced hypercholesterolemia in a transgenic mouse model of Alzheimer disease. Neurobiol Dis. 2004;16:124–132.

Gillardon F, Bottiger B, Schmitz B, Zimmermann M, Hossmann KA.

Activation of CPP-32 protease in hippocampal neurons following ischemia and epilepsy. Brain Res Mol Brain Res. 1997;50:16–22.

Grant WB. Dietary links to Alzheimer's disease: 1999 update. J Alzheimers Dis. 1999;1:197–201.
33   Greene AE, Todorova MT, McGowan R, Seyfried TN. Caloric restriction inhibits seizure susceptibility in epileptic EL mice by reducing blood glucose. Epilepsia. 2001;42:1371–1378.

Hashimoto M, Hossain S, Shimada T, Sugioka K, Yamasaki H, Fujii Y, et al. Docosahexaenoic acid provides protection from impairment of learning ability in Alzheimer's disease model rats. J Neurochem. 2002;81:1084–1091.

Hashimoto M, Tanabe Y, Fujii Y, Kikuta T, Shibata H, Shido O. Chronic administration of docosahexaenoic acid ameliorates the impairment of spatial cognition learning ability in amyloid β-infused rats. J Nutr. 2005;135:549–555.

Hemingway C, Freeman JM, Pillas DJ, Pyzik PL. The ketogenic diet: a 3- to 6- year follow-up of 150 children enrolled prospectively. Pediatrics. 2001;108:898–905.

Henderson ST. High carbohydrate diets and Alzheimer's disease. Med Hypotheses. 2004;62:689–700.

Ho L, Qin W, Pompl PN, Xiang Z, Wang J, Zhao Z, et al. Diet-induced insulin resistance promotes amyloidosis in a transgenic mouse model of Alzheimer's disease. FASEB J. 2004;18:902–904.

Holmer HK, Keyghobadi M, Moore C, Menashe RA, Meshul CK. Dietary restriction affects striatal glutamate in the MPTP-induced mouse model of nigrostriatal degeneration. Synapse. 2005;57:100–112.

Hori A, Tandon P, Holmes GL, Stafstrom CE. Ketogenic diet: effects on expression of kindled seizures and behavior in adult rats. Epilepsia. 1997;38:750–758.

Huttenlocher PR. Ketonemia and seizures: metabolic and anticonvulsant effects of two ketogenic diets in childhood epilepsy. Pediatr Res. 1976;10:536–540.

Huttenlocher PR, Wilbourn AJ, Signore JM. Medium-chain triglycerides as a therapy for intractable childhood epilepsy. Neurology. 1971;21:1097–1103.

Jones SE, Jomary C. Clusterin. Int J Biochem Cell Biol. 2002;34:427–431.

Kalmijn S, Launer LJ, Ott A, Witteman JC, Hofman A, Breteler MM. Dietary fat intake and the risk of incident dementia in the Rotterdam Study. Ann Neurol. 1997;42:776–782.

Kashiwaya Y, Takeshima T, Mori N, Nakashima K, Clarke K, Veech RL. d-β-hydroxybutyrate protects neurons in models of Alzheimer's and Parkinson's disease. Proc Natl Acad Sci USA. 2000;97:5440–5444.

Kossoff EH. More fat and fewer seizures: dietary therapies for epilepsy. Lancet Neurol. 2004;3:415–420.

Kossoff EH, McGrogan JR, Bluml RM, Pillas DJ, Rubenstein JE, Vining EP. A modified atkins diet is effective for the treatment of intractable pediatric epilepsy. Epilepsia. 2006;47:421–424.

Lee J, Bruce-Keller AJ, Kruman Y, Chan SL, Mattson MP. 2-Deoxy-d-glucose protects hippocampal neurons against excitotoxic and oxidative injury: evidence for the involvement of stress proteins. J Neurosci Res. 1999;57:48–61.

Lee J, Kim SJ, Son TG, Chan SL, Mattson MP. Interferon-gamma is upregulated in the hippocampus in response to intermittent fasting and protects hippocampal neurons against excitotoxicity. J Neurosci Res. 2006;83:1552–1557.

Levin-Allerhand JA, Lominska CE, Smith JD. Increased amyloid-levels in APPSWE transgenic mice treated chronically with a physiological high-fat high-cholesterol diet. J Nutr Health Aging. 2002;6:315–319.

Likhodii SS, Musa K, Mendonca A, Dell C, Burnham WM, Cunnane SC. Dietary fat, ketosis, and seizure resistance in rats on the ketogenic diet. Epilepsia. 2000;41:1400–1410.

Lim GP, Calon F, Morihara T, Yang F, Teter B, Ubeda O, et al. A diet enriched with the omega-3 fatty acid docosahexaenoic acid reduces amyloid burden in an aged Alzheimer mouse model. J Neurosci. 2005;25:3032–3040.

Mantis JG, Centeno NA, Todorova MT, McGowan R, Seyfried TN. Management of multifactorial idiopathic epilepsy in EL mice with caloric restriction and the ketogenic diet: role of glucose and ketone bodies. Nutr Metab (London) 2004;1:11.

Marie C, Bralet AM, Gueldry S, Bralet J. Fasting prior to transient cerebral ischemia reduces delayed neuronal necrosis. Metab Brain Dis. 1990;5:65–75.

Marsh EB, Freeman JM, Kossoff EH, Vining EP, Rubenstein JE, Pyzik PL, Hemingway C. The outcome of children with intractable seizures: a 3- to 6-year follow-up of 67 children who remained on the ketogenic diet less than one year. Epilepsia. 2006;47:425–430.

Massieu L, Del RP, Montiel T. Neurotoxicity of glutamate uptake inhibition in vivo: correlation with succinate dehydrogenase activity and prevention by energy substrates. Neuroscience. 2001;106:669–677.

Massieu L, Haces ML, Montiel T, Hernandez-Fonseca K. Acetoacetate protects hippocampal neurons against glutamate-mediated neuronal damage during glycolysis inhibition. Neuroscience. 2003;120:365–378.

Maswood N, Young J, Tilmont E, Zhang Z, Gash DM, Gerhardt GA, et al. Caloric restriction increases neurotrophic factor levels and attenuates neurochemical and behavioral deficits in a primate model of Parkinson's disease. Proc Natl Acad Sci USA. 2004;101:18171–18176.

Mattson MP, Cheng B, Baldwin SA, Smith-Swintosky VL, Keller J, Geddes JW, et al. Brain injury and tumor necrosis factors induce calbindin D-28k in astrocytes: evidence for a cytoprotective response. J Neurosci Res. 1995;42:357–370.

McIntosh TK, Saatman KE, Raghupathi R, Graham DI, Smith DH, Lee VM, Trojanowski JQ. The Dorothy Russell Memorial Lecture. The molecular and cellular sequelae of experimental traumatic brain injury: pathogenetic mechanisms. Neuropathol Appl Neurobiol. 1998;24:251–267.

Morris MC, Evans DA, Bienias JL, Tangney CC, Bennett DA, Aggarwal N, et al. Dietary fats and the risk of incident Alzheimer disease. Arch Neurol. 2003a;60:194–200.

Morris MC, Evans DA, Bienias JL, Tangney CC, Bennett DA, Wilson RS, et al. Consumption of fish and n-3 fatty acids and risk of incident Alzheimer disease. Arch Neurol. 2003b;60:940–946.

Morris MC, Evans DA, Bienias JL, Tangney CC, Wilson RS. Dietary fat intake and 6-year cognitive change in an older biracial community population. Neurology. 2004;62:1573–1579.

Muller-Schwarze AB, Tandon P, Liu Z, Yang Y, Holmes GL, Stafstrom CE. Ketogenic diet reduces spontaneous seizures and mossy fiber sprouting in the kainic acid model. Neuroreport. 1999;10:1517–1522.

Musa-Veloso K, Likhodii SS, Cunnane SC. Breath acetone is a reliable indicator of ketosis in adults consuming ketogenic meals. Am J Clin Nutr. 2002;76:65–70.

Nehlig A. Brain uptake and metabolism of ketone bodies in animal models. Prostaglandins Leukot Essent Fatty Acids. 2004;70:265–275.

Neuroinflammation Working Group. Inflammation and Alzheimer's disease. Neurobiol Aging. 2000;21:383–421.

Noh HS, Kim YS, Lee HP, Chung KM, Kim DW, Kang SS, et al. The protective effect of a ketogenic diet on kainic acid-induced hippocampal cell death in the male ICR mice. Epilepsy Res. 2003;53:119–128.

Noh HS, Kang SS, Kim DW, Kim YH, Park CH, Han JY, et al. Ketogenic diet increases calbindin-D28k in the hippocampi of male ICR mice with kainic acid seizures. Epilepsy Res. 2005a;65:153–159.

Noh HS, Kim DW, Kang SS, Cho GJ, Choi WS. Ketogenic diet prevents clusterin accumulation induced by kainic acid in the hippocampus of male ICR mice. Brain Res. 2005b;1042:114–118.

Noh HS, Hah YS, Nilufar R, Han J, Bong JH, Kang SS, et al. Acetoacetate protects neuronal cells from oxidative glutamate toxicity. J Neurosci Res. 2006;83:702–709. [PubMed]

Palmblad J, Hafstrom I, Ringertz B. Antirheumatic effects of fasting. Rheum Dis Clin North Am. 1991;17:351–362.

Pan JW, de Graaf RA, Petersen KF, Shulman GI, Hetherington HP, Rothman DL. [2,4-13C2]-β-Hydroxybutyrate metabolism in human brain. J Cereb Blood Flow Metab. 2002;22:890–898.

Patel NV, Gordon MN, Connor KE, Good RA, Engelman RW, Mason J, et al. Caloric restriction attenuates Aβ-deposition in Alzheimer transgenic models. Neurobiol Aging. 2005;26:995–1000.

Pierre K, Pellerin L. Monocarboxylate transporters in the central nervous system: distribution, regulation and function. J Neurochem. 2005;94:1–14.

Pratico D, Trojanowski JQ. Inflammatory hypotheses: novel mechanisms of Alzheimer's neurodegeneration and new therapeutic targets? Neurobiol Aging. 2000;21:441–445.

Prins ML, Lee SM, Fujima LS, Hovda DA. Increased cerebral uptake and oxidation of exogenous βHB improves ATP following traumatic brain injury in adult rats. J Neurochem. 2004;90:666–672.

Prins ML, Fujima LS, Hovda DA. Age-dependent reduction of cortical contusion volume by ketones after traumatic brain injury. J Neurosci Res. 2005;82:413–420.

Rafiki A, Boulland JL, Halestrap AP, Ottersen OP, Bergersen L. Highly differential expression of the monocarboxylate transporters MCT2 and MCT4 in the developing rat brain. Neuroscience. 2003;122:677–688.

Reger MA, Henderson ST, Hale C, Cholerton B, Baker LD, Watson GS, et al. Effects of β-hydroxybutyrate on cognition in memory-impaired adults. Neurobiol Aging. 2004;25:311–314.

Rho JM, Anderson GD, Donevan SD, White HS. Acetoacetate, acetone, and dibenzylamine (a contaminant in L-(+)-β-hydroxybutyrate) exhibit direct anticonvulsant actions *in vivo*. Epilepsia. 2002;43:358–361.

Ruitenberg A, Kalmijn S, de Ridder MA, Redekop WK, van HF, Hofman A, et al. Prognosis of Alzheimer's disease: the Rotterdam Study. Neuroepidemiology. 2001;20:188–195.

Schachter SC. Current evidence indicates that antiepileptic drugs are anti-ictal, not antiepileptic. Epilepsy Res. 2002;50:67–70.

Schwartz RH, Eaton J, Bower BD, ynsley-Green A. Ketogenic diets in the treatment of epilepsy: short-term clinical effects. Dev Med Child Neurol. 1989;31:145–151.

Shie FS, Jin LW, Cook DG, Leverenz JB, LeBoeuf RC. Diet-induced hypercholesterolemia enhances brain Aβ accumulation in transgenic mice. Neuroreport. 2002;13:455–459.

Sinha SR, Kossoff EH. The ketogenic diet. Neurologist. 2005;11:161–170.

Smith SL, Heal DJ, Martin KF. KTX 0101: a potential metabolic approach to cytoprotection in major surgery and neurological disorders. CNS Drug Rev. 2005;11:113–140.

Stafstrom CE. Animal models of the ketogenic diet: what have we learned, what can we learn? Epilepsy Res. 1999;37:241–259.

Stafstrom CE. Dietary approaches to epilepsy treatment: old and new options on the menu. Epilepsy Curr. 2004;4:215–222.

Stafstrom CE, Wang C, Jensen FE. Electrophysiological observations in hippocampal slices from rats treated with the ketogenic diet. Dev Neurosci. 1999;21:393–399.

Stamp LK, James MJ, Cleland LG. Diet and rheumatoid arthritis: a review of the literature. Semin Arthritis Rheum. 2005;35:77–94.

Su SW, Cilio MR, Sogawa Y, Silveira DC, Holmes GL, Stafstrom CE. Timing of ketogenic diet initiation in an experimental epilepsy model. Brain Res Dev Brain Res. 2000;125:131–138.

Sullivan PG, Rippy NA, Dorenbos K, Concepcion RC, Agarwal AK, Rho JM. The ketogenic diet increases mitochondrial uncoupling protein levels and activity. Ann Neurol. 2004;55:576–580.

Suzuki M, Suzuki M, Sato K, Dohi S, Sato T, Matsuura A, Hiraide A. Effect of β-hydroxybutyrate, a cerebral function improving agent, on cerebral hypoxia, anoxia and ischemia in mice and rats. Jpn J Pharmacol. 2001;87:143–150.

Suzuki M, Suzuki M, Kitamura Y, Mori S, Sato K, Dohi S, et al. β-hydroxybutyrate, a cerebral function improving agent, protects rat brain against ischemic damage caused by permanent and transient focal cerebral ischemia. Jpn J Pharmacol. 2002;89:36–43.

Thavendiranathan P, Mendonca A, Dell C, Likhodii SS, Musa K, Iracleous C, et al. The MCT ketogenic diet: effects on animal seizure models. Exp Neurol. 2000;161:696–703.

Thavendiranathan P, Chow C, Cunnane S, McIntyre BW. The effect of the 'classic' ketogenic diet on animal seizure models. Brain Res. 2003;959:206–213.

Tieu K, Perier C, Caspersen C, Teismann P, Wu DC, Yan SD, et al. d-β-hydroxybutyrate rescues mitochondrial respiration and mitigates features of Parkinson disease. J Clin Invest. 2003;112:892–901.

Todorova MT, Tandon P, Madore RA, Stafstrom CE, Seyfried TN. The ketogenic diet inhibits epileptogenesis in EL mice: a genetic model for idiopathic epilepsy. Epilepsia. 2000;41:933–940.

Trevathan E. Infantile spasms and Lennox-Gastaut syndrome. J Child Neurol. 2002;17 Suppl 2:2S9–2S22.

Van der Auwera I, Wera S, Van LF, Henderson ST. A ketogenic diet reduces amyloid beta 40 and 42 in a mouse model of Alzheimer's disease. Nutr Metab (London) 2005;2:28.

VanItallie TB, Nonas C, Di RA, Boyar K, Hyams K, Heymsfield SB. Treatment of Parkinson disease with diet-induced hyperketonemia: a feasibility study. Neurology. 2005;64:728–730.

Vannucci SJ, Simpson IA. Developmental switch in brain nutrient transporter expression in the rat. Am J Physiol Endocrinol Metab. 2003;285:E1127–E1134.

Veech RL. The therapeutic implications of ketone bodies: the effects of ketone bodies in pathological conditions: ketosis, ketogenic diet, redox states, insulin resistance, and mitochondrial metabolism. Prostaglandins Leukot Essent Fatty Acids. 2004;70:309–319.

Veech RL, Chance B, Kashiwaya Y, Lardy HA, Cahill GF., Jr Ketone bodies, potential therapeutic uses. IUBMB Life. 2001;51:241–247.

Vezzani A, Granata T. Brain inflammation in epilepsy: experimental and clinical evidence. Epilepsia. 2005;46:1724–1743.

Vining EP, Freeman JM, Ballaban-Gil K, Camfield CS, Camfield PR,

Holmes GL, et al. A multicenter study of the efficacy of the ketogenic diet. Arch Neurol. 1998;55:1433–1437.

Wang ZJ, Bergqvist C, Hunter JV, Jin D, Wang DJ, Wehrli S, Zimmerman RA. *In vivo* measurement of brain metabolites using two-dimensional double-quantum MR spectroscopy: exploration of GABA levels in a ketogenic diet. Magn Reson Med. 2003;49:615–619.

Wang J, Ho L, Qin W, Rocher AB, Seror I, Humala N, et al. Caloric restriction attenuates β-amyloid neuropathology in a mouse model of Alzheimer's disease. FASEB J. 2005;19:659–661.

Wilder RM. The effects of ketonemia on the course of epilepsy. Mayo Clin Proc. 1921;2:307–308.

Yamada KA, Rensing N, Thio LL. Ketogenic diet reduces hypoglycemia-induced neuronal death in young rats. Neurosci Lett. 2005;385:210–214.

Young KW, Greenwood CE, van RR, Binns MA. A randomized, crossover trial of high-carbohydrate foods in nursing home residents with Alzheimer's disease: associations among intervention response, body mass index, and behavioral and cognitive function. J Gerontol A Biol Sci Med Sci. 2005;60:1039–1045.

Yudkoff M, Daikhin Y, Nissim I, Lazarow A, Nissim I. Ketogenic diet, amino acid metabolism, and seizure control. J Neurosci Res. 2001;66:931–940.

Ziegler DR, Ribeiro LC, Hagenn M, Siqueira IR, Araujo E, Torres IL, et al. Ketogenic diet increases glutathione peroxidase activity in rat hippocampus. Neurochem Res. 2003;28:1793–1797.

Fatty liver disease

Fox CS, Coady S, Sorlie PD, et al. Increasing cardiovascular disease burden due to diabetes mellitus: the Framingham Heart Study. Circulation. 2007;115(12):1544–50.

Flegal KM, Carroll MD, Ogden CL, Curtin LR. Prevalence and trends in obesity among US adults, 1999–
2008. JAMA. 2010;303(3):235–41. Overall, obesity affects 35.5% and 35.8% of U.S. men and women, respectively. This study of 5555 patients examines the prevalence of obesity in the population according to age and ethnicity.

Brookheart RT, Michel CI, Schaffer JE. As a matter of fat. Cell Metab. 2009;10(1):9–12.
Fabbrini E, Magkos F, Mohammed BS, et al. Intrahepatic fat, not visceral fat, is linked with metabolic complications of obesity. Proc Natl Acad Sci U S A. 2009;106(36):15430–5.
Brunt EM. Pathology of nonalcoholic fatty liver disease. Nat Rev Gastroenterol Hepatol. 2010;7(4):195–203. Study focuses on the state-of-the-art histological hallmarks of NAFLD disease progression.

Fabbrini E, Sullivan S, Klein S. Obesity and nonalcoholic fatty liver disease: biochemical, metabolic, and clinical implications. Hepatology. 2010;51(2):679–89.Outstanding review highlights the relationship between NAFLD pathogenesis and metabolic dysfunction.

York LW, Puthalapattu S, Wu GY. Nonalcoholic fatty liver disease and low-carbohydrate diets. Annu Rev Nutr. 2009;29:365–79.

Best TH, Franz DN, Gilbert DL, et al. Cardiac complications in pediatric patients on the ketogenic diet. Neurology. 2000;54(12):2328–30.

Chen TY, Smith W, Rosenstock JL, Lessnau KD. A life-threatening complication of Atkins diet. Lancet. 2006;367(9514):958.

Tiniakos DG, Vos MB, Brunt EM. Nonalcoholic fatty liver disease: pathology and pathogenesis. Annu Rev Pathol. 2010;5:145–71.

Cohen JC, Horton JD, Hobbs HH. Human fatty liver disease: old questions and new insights. Science. 2011;332(6037):1519–23.Timely review focusing on the recent mechanistic insights into human

NAFLD.

Sunny NE, Parks EJ, Browning JD, Burgess SC. Excessive Hepatic Mitochondrial TCA Cycle and Gluconeogenesis in Humans with Nonalcoholic Fatty Liver Disease. Cell Metab. 2011;14(6):804–10. Powerful study using MRS and NMR in human NAFLD demonstrating metabolic differences between NAFLD and healthy patients, which indicates a link between increased oxidative metabolism, gluconeogenesis, and anaplerosis in IHTG.

Maher JJ. New insights from rodent models of fatty liver disease. Antioxid Redox Signal. 2011;15(2):535–50. Focuses on the genetic and dietary mouse models used to investigate the pathologies of NAFLD.

Tetri LH, Basaranoglu M, Brunt EM, et al. Severe NAFLD with hepatic necroinflammatory changes in mice fed trans fats and a high-fructose corn syrup equivalent. Am J Physiol Gastrointest Liver Physiol. 2008;295(5):G987–95.
15. Koppe SW, Elias M, Moseley RH, Green RM. Trans fat feeding results in higher serum alanine aminotransferase and increased insulin resistance compared with a standard murine high-fat diet. Am J Physiol Gastrointest Liver Physiol. 2009;297(2):G378–84.

Sullivan S. Implications of diet on nonalcoholic fatty liver disease. Curr Opin Gastroenterol. 2010;26(2):160–4.

Dhibi M, Brahmi F, Mnari A, et al. The intake of high fat diet with different trans fatty acid levels differentially induces oxidative stress and non alcoholic fatty liver disease (NAFLD) in rats. Nutr Metab (Lond) 2011;8(1):65.

Marsman HA, Heger M, Kloek JJ, et al. Reversal of hepatic steatosis by omega-3 fatty acids measured non-invasively by (1) H-magnetic resonance spectroscopy in a rat model.J Gastroenterol Hepatol. 2011;26(2):356–63.

Nagai Y, Yonemitsu S, Erion DM, et al. The role of peroxisome proliferator-activated receptor gamma coactivator-1 beta in the

pathogenesis of fructose-induced insulin resistance. Cell Metab. 2009;9(3):252–64. In addition to the improvements in glucose homeostasis, the authors demonstrate that reducing PGC-1β expression is sufficient to prevent increased IHTG deposition during a high fructose feeding
.

Pickens MK, Yan JS, Ng RK, et al. Dietary sucrose is essential to the development of liver injury in the methionine-choline-deficient model of steatohepatitis. J Lipid Res.2009;50(10):2072–82. Demonstrates that MCD diet-induced NAFLD is dependent on simple sugars – MCD diet that incorporates starch, rather than sucrose, markedly attenuates NAFLD signatures

Pickens MK, Ogata H, Soon RK, et al. Dietary fructose exacerbates hepatocellular injury when incorporated into a methionine-choline-deficient diet. Liver Int.2010;30(8):1229–39.

Corbin KD, Zeisel SH. Choline metabolism provides novel insights into nonalcoholic fatty liver disease and its progression. Curr Opin Gastroenterol. 2011

Caballero F, Fernandez A, Matias N, et al. Specific contribution of methionine and choline in nutritional nonalcoholic steatohepatitis: impact on mitochondrial S-adenosyl-L-methionine and glutathione. J Biol Chem. 2010;285(24):18528–36. Study segregates the effects of methionine deficiency and choline deficiency in the promotion of NAFLD. Methionine deficiency leads to hepatocellular injury, oxidative stress and inflammation, while choline deficiency is primarily responsible for increased IHTG.

McGarry JD, Foster DW. Regulation of hepatic fatty acid oxidation and ketone body production. Annu Rev Biochem. 1980;49:395–420. Classical review written by pioneers of the regulation of hepatic fatty acid oxidation and ketogenesis.

Shimazu T, Hirschey MD, Hua L, et al. SIRT3 Deacetylates Mitochondrial 3-Hydroxy-3-Methylglutaryl CoA Synthase 2 and Regulates Ketone Body Production. Cell Metab. 2010;12(6):654–61.

Sengupta S, Peterson TR, Laplante M, et al. mTORC1 controls fasting-induced ketogenesis and its modulation by ageing. Nature. 2010;468(7327):1100–4.

Cotter DG, d'Avignon DA, Wentz AE, et al. Obligate role for ketone body oxidation in neonatal metabolic homeostasis. J Biol Chem. 2011;286(9):6902–6910.

Kossoff EH, Hartman AL. Ketogenic diets: new advances for metabolism-based therapies. Curr Opin Neurol. 2012;25(2):173–8.

Yang X, Cheng B. Neuroprotective and anti-inflammatory activities of ketogenic diet on MPTP-induced neurotoxicity. J Mol Neurosci. 2010;42(2):145–53.

Yao J, Chen S, Mao Z, et al. 2-Deoxy-D-glucose treatment induces ketogenesis, sustains mitochondrial function, and reduces pathology in female mouse model of Alzheimer's disease. PLoS One. 2011;6(7):e21788.

Seyfried TN, Kiebish MA, Marsh J, et al. Metabolic management of brain cancer.Biochim Biophys Acta. 2011;1807(6):577–94.

McNally MA, Hartman AL. Ketone Bodies in Epilepsy. J Neurochem.2012;121(1):28–35.

Patel A, Pyzik PL, Turner Z, et al. Long-term outcomes of children treated with the ketogenic diet in the past. Epilepsia. 2010;51(7):1277–82.

Zeng LH, Rensing NR, Wong M. The mammalian target of rapamycin signaling pathway mediates epileptogenesis in a model of temporal lobe epilepsy. J Neurosci.2009;29(21):6964–72.

McDaniel SS, Wong M. Therapeutic role of mammalian target of rapamycin (mTOR) inhibition in preventing epileptogenesis. Neurosci Lett. 2011;497(3):231–9.]

Thio LL. Hypothalamic hormones and metabolism. Epilepsy

Res. 2011 Epub ahead of print.

Sharma S, Gulati S. The ketogenic diet and the QT interval. J Clin Neurosci.2012;19(1):181–2.

Browning JD, Baker JA, Rogers T, et al. Short-term weight loss and hepatic triglyceride reduction: evidence of a metabolic advantage with dietary carbohydrate restriction. Am J Clin Nutr. 2011;93(5):1048–52. A small clinical trial that suggests that short-term carbohydrate restriction is more efficacious at reducing IHTG than caloric restriction. Patients on the low-carbohydrate diet had decreased respiratory quotients and increased plasma ketone levels, suggesting the decreased IHTG was achieved through increased hepatic mitochondrial β-oxidation.

Foster GD, Wyatt HR, Hill JO, et al. Weight and metabolic outcomes after 2 years on a low-carbohydrate versus low-fat diet: a randomized trial. Ann Intern Med.2010;153(3):147–Over two years, both low-fat and low-carbohydrate diets both promoted weight loss in a randomized trial of 307 patients. However, the use of low-carbohydrate diets also led to decreases in blood pressure and serum triglycerides, VLDL and LDL levels and increases in HDL, suggesting that low-carbohydrate diets can reduce cardiovascular disease risk factors

Kennedy AR, Pissios P, Otu H, et al. A high-fat, ketogenic diet induces a unique metabolic state in mice. Am J Physiol Endocrinol Metab. 2007;292(6):E1724–39.Describes the unique metabolic effects of the commonly-used Bio-Serv F3666 ketogenic diet in mice.

Garbow JR, Doherty JM, Schugar RC, et al. Hepatic steatosis, inflammation, and ER stress in mice maintained long term on a very low-carbohydrate ketogenic diet. Am J Physiol Gastrointest Liver Physiol. 2011;300(6):G956–67. This study compares and contrasts the long-term effects of a high-simple sugar, high-fat Western diet to the very low-carbohydrate, high-fat ketogenic diet (Bio-Serv F3666) on NAFLD signatures in mice. Ketogenic diet-fed mice ultimately develop NAFLD and systemic glucose intolerance, but whole-body insulin responsiveness was not impaired.

Bielohuby M, Menhofer D, Kirchner H, et al. Induction of ketosis in rats fed low-carbohydrate, high fat diets depends on the relative abundance of dietary fat and protein.Am J Physiol Endocrinol Metab. 2011;300:E65–E76.
Goettsch M. Comparative protein requirement of the rat and mouse for growth, reproduction and lactation using casein diets. J Nutr. 1960;70:307–12.

Berglund ED, Li CY, Bina HA, et al. Fibroblast growth factor 21 controls glycemia via regulation of hepatic glucose flux and insulin sensitivity. Endocrinology.2009;150(9):4084–93.

Fisher FM, Estall JL, Adams AC, et al. Integrated regulation of hepatic metabolism by fibroblast growth factor 21 (FGF21) in vivo. Endocrinology. 2011;152(8):2996–3004.

Badman MK, Koester A, Flier JS, et al. Fibroblast growth factor 21-deficient mice demonstrate impaired adaptation to ketosis. Endocrinology. 2009;150(11):4931–40.

Fisher FM, Chui PC, Antonellis PJ, et al. Obesity is a fibroblast growth factor 21 (FGF21)-resistant state. Diabetes. 2010;59(11):2781–9.

Domouzoglou EM, Maratos-Flier E. Fibroblast growth factor 21 is a metabolic regulator that plays a role in the adaptation to ketosis. Am J Clin Nutr. 2011;93(4):901S–5.

Badman MK, Kennedy AR, Adams AC, et al. A Very Low Carbohydrate Ketogenic Diet Improves Glucose Tolerance in ob/ob Mice Independent of Weight Loss. Am J Physiol Endocrinol Metab. 2009;297:E1197–E1204.

Jornayvaz FR, Jurczak MJ, Lee HY, et al. A high-fat, ketogenic diet causes hepatic insulin resistance in mice despite increasing energy expenditure and preventing weight gain. Am J Physiol Endocrinol Metab. 2010;299(5):E808–15. In contradiction to other studies using Bio-Serv F3666 ketogenic diet, this study finds that KD-feeding leads to hepatic insulin resistance, and links this to increased hepatic DAG and PKCε activation.

McGuinness OP, Ayala JE, Laughlin MR, Wasserman DH. NIH experiment in centralized mouse phenotyping: the Vanderbilt experience and recommendations for evaluating glucose homeostasis in the mouse. Am J Physiol Endocrinol Metab.2009;297(4):E849–55. Carefully evaluates the merits and limitations of glucose and insulin tolerance tests, and hyperinsulinemic-euglycemic clamp studies in mice.

Monetti M, Levin MC, Watt MJ, et al. Hepatic acyl-CoA:diacylglcyerol acyltransferase (DGAT) overexpression, diacylglycerol, and insulin sensitivity. Proc Natl Acad Sci U S A. 2011;108(34):E523. author reply E524.

ABOUT THE AUTHORS

Roderick is in his 60s and has been practicing natural medicine for the last 37 years in London and Jersey, He studied at the Howell College, Shen Doa Institute and also studied Classical Chinese Medicine as part of his martial arts training.

Roderick specialises in endocrine issues and fertility. Endocrine issues can cover a multitude of problems and symptoms from PMT, menopause, peri-menopause on to such things as hypoglycemia and thyroid disorders.

He is the co-founder of the London College of Naturopathic medicine, which is acknowledged as offering one of the best Naturopathic training tuitions in Europe.

He has a keen interest in natural product design and have designed products for several of the leading nutrition companies within the UK. He designed the award-winning and best-selling products Spectrumzyme, Polyzymeforte and GI-Complex.

Elizabeth Bright is in her 50s. She is married, with three children She is a certified Osteopath and Naturopath practicing in Sanremo, Italy. She studied at Columbia University in New York City where she majored in Oriental and Central Asian Studies. This took her to China where she lived for two years. Her studies continued to include Classical Chinese medicine and bonesetting to complement her martial arts training. She is a fourth generation master of Chau Ka Kung Fu. Elizabeth was chef/owner of two award-winning organic restaurants in Washington, DC. She speaks regularly on women's health issues and is the guest Naturopath on Mi Presento, Sono Donna! a television show dedicated to educating women about natural health. Elizabeth speaks Italian, French, German, Spanish, and Mandarin.